T0358924

Treatment of Acute and Chronic Tendon Rupture and Tendinopathy

Editor

SELENE G. PAREKH

FOOT AND ANKLE CLINICS

www.foot.theclinics.com

Consulting Editor
MARK S. MYERSON

December 2017 • Volume 22 • Number 4

ELSEVIER

1600 John F. Kennedy Boulevard ● Suite 1800 ● Philadelphia, Pennsylvania, 19103-2899

http://www.theclinics.com

FOOT AND ANKLE CLINICS Volume 22, Number 4
December 2017 ISSN 1083-7515, ISBN-13: 978-0-323-55276-9

Editor: Lauren Boyle
Developmental Editor: Meredith Madeira

Foot and Ankle Clinics (ISSN 1083-7515) is published quarterly by Elsevier, Inc., 360 Park Avenue South, New York, NY 10010-1710. Months of issue are March, June, September, and December. Periodicals postage paid at New York, NY, and additional mailing offices. Subscription price per year is $320.00 (US individuals), $489.00 (US institutions), $100.00 (US students), $360.00 (Canadian individuals), $588.00 (Canadian institutions), $215.00 (Canadian students), $460.00 (international individuals), $588.00 (international institutions), and $215.00 (international students). To receive student/resident rate, orders must be accompanied by name of affiliated institution, date of term, and the *signature* of program/residency coordinator on institution letterhead. Orders will be billed at individual rate until proof of status is received. Foreign air speed delivery is included in all *Clinics* subscription prices. All prices are subject to change without notice. **POSTMASTER:** Send address changes to *Foot and Ankle Clinics*, Elsevier Health Sciences Division, Subscription Customer Service, 3251 Riverport Lane, Maryland Heights, MO 63043. **Customer Service: 1-800-654-2452 (US and Canada). From outside of the United States and Canada, call 314-447-8871. Fax: 314-447-8029. E-mail: JournalsCustomerService-usa@ elsevier.com (for print support); JournalsOnlineSupport-usa@elsevier.com (for online support).**

Reprints. For copies of 100 or more, of articles in this publication, please contact the Commercial Reprints Department, Elsevier Inc., 360 Park Avenue South, New York, NY 10010-1710. Tel.: 212-633-3874; Fax: 212-633-3820; E-mail: reprints@elsevier.com.

Contributors

CONSULTING EDITOR

MARK S. MYERSON, MD
Medical Director, The Foot and Ankle Association, Inc, Baltimore, Maryland, USA

EDITOR

SELENE G. PAREKH, MD, MBA, FAOA
Partner, North Carolina Orthopaedic Clinic, Professor, Department of Orthopaedic Surgery, Adjunct Faculty, Fuqua School of Business, Duke University, Durham, North Carolina, USA

AUTHORS

SAMUEL B. ADAMS, MD
Foot and Ankle Division, Department of Orthopedic Surgery, Duke University Medical Center, Durham, North Carolina, USA

ANNUNZIATO AMENDOLA, MD
Professor, Duke University Medical Center, Durham, North Carolina, USA

DAVID BECK, MD
Chief Resident, Department of Orthopaedic Surgery, Thomas Jefferson University, The Rothman Institute, Bryn Mawr, Pennsylvania

GREGORY C. BERLET, MD
Orthopedic Surgeon, The Orthopedic Foot & Ankle Center, Westerville, Ohio, USA

JAMES W. BRODSKY, MD
Director, Foot and Ankle Surgery Fellowship Program, Baylor University Medical Center, Professor of Surgery, Orthopaedics, Texas A&M College of Medicine, Clinical Professor of Orthopaedic Surgery, The University of Texas Southwestern Medical Center, Dallas, Texas, USA

ARASH CALAFI, MD
Resident, Department of Orthopaedic Surgery, University of California, Davis, Sacramento, California, USA

REBECCA CERRATO, MD
Orthopaedic Surgeon, Mercy Medical Center, Foot and Ankle Surgery Fellowship Director, Institute for Foot and Ankle Reconstruction, Baltimore, Maryland, USA

CHRISTOPHER P. CHIODO, MD
Foot and Ankle Division Chief, Department of Orthopaedic Surgery, Brigham and Women's Hospital, Boston, Massachusetts, USA

BRUCE COHEN, MD
OrthoCarolina Foot and Ankle Institute, Charlotte, North Carolina, USA

TRAVIS J. DEKKER, MD
Foot and Ankle Division, Department of Orthopedic Surgery, Duke University Medical Center, Durham, North Carolina, USA

CHRIS DIEFENBACH, MD
Foot and Ankle Surgery, Department of Orthopaedic Surgery, University of California, Davis, Sacramento, California, USA

ANDREW E. FEDERER, MD
Foot and Ankle Division, Department of Orthopedic Surgery, Duke University Medical Center, Durham, North Carolina, USA

ERIC GIZA, MD
Chief, Foot and Ankle Surgery, Department of Orthopaedic Surgery, University of California, Davis, Sacramento, California, USA

CHRISTOPHER E. GROSS, MD
Assistant Professor, Department of Orthopaedics, Medical University of South Carolina, Charleston, South Carolina, USA

KAMRAN S. HAMID, MD, MPH
Assistant Professor, Rush University Medical Center, Chicago, Illinois, USA

ELIZABETH HARKIN, MD
Resident Physician, Department of Orthopaedic Surgery and Rehabilitation, Loyola University Medical Center, Maywood, Illinois, USA

JUSTIN M. KANE, MD
Orthopaedic Surgeon, Foot and Ankle Surgery Division, Baylor University Medical Center, Clinical Professor, Texas A&M University Health Science Center, Dallas, Texas, USA

CHRIS KREULEN, MD
Foot and Ankle Surgery, Department of Orthopaedics, University of California, Davis, Sacramento, California, USA

JORDAN L. LILES, MD
Foot and Ankle Division, Department of Orthopedic Surgery, Duke University Medical Center, Durham, North Carolina, USA

JAMES A. NUNLEY, MD
Professor, Department of Orthopaedic Surgery, Duke University Medical Center, Durham, North Carolina, USA

SAMPAT DUMBRE PATIL, DNB (Orth)
Orthopaedic Foot and Ankle Surgeon, President, Indian Foot and Ankle Society, Director, Noble Hospital, Pune, India

DAVID PEDOWITZ, MS, MD
Associate Professor, Department of Orthopaedic Surgery, Thomas Jefferson University, Foot and Ankle Division, The Rothman Institute, Bryn Mawr, Pennsylvania; Consulting Physician, Philadelphia Phillies, Philadelphia 76ers, Philadelphia, USA

MICHAEL PINZUR, MD
Professor and Quality Medical Director, Department of Orthopaedic Surgery and Rehabilitation, Loyola University Medical Center, Maywood, Illinois, USA

STEVEN M. RAIKIN, MD
Professor of Orthopaedic Surgery, Director, Foot and Ankle Service, Rothman Institute at Jefferson, Sidney Kimmel Medical College, Philadelphia, Pennsylvania, USA

ADAM SCHIFF, MD
Assistant Professor, Associate Program Director, Department of Orthopaedic Surgery and Rehabilitation, Loyola University Medical Center, Maywood, Illinois, USA

OLIVER SCHIPPER, MD
OrthoCarolina Foot and Ankle Institute, Charlotte, North Carolina, USA; Anderson Orthopaedic Clinic, Arlington, Virginia, USA

RAJIV SHAH, MS
Orthopaedic Foot and Ankle Surgeon, Executive Board Member, Global Foot and Ankle Council, Vice Chairman, Asia-Pacific Foot and Ankle Council, South Asia Corodinator and International Advisory Board Member, Foot Innovate International Webinars Past President, Indian Foot and Ankle Society, Managing Director, Sunshine Global Hospitals, Vadodara, Gujarat, India; Managing Director, Sunshine Global Hospitals, Bharuch, Gujarat, India; Managing Director, Sunshine Global Hospitals, Surat, Gujarat, India

RACHEL J. SHAKKED, MD
Assistant Professor of Orthopaedic Surgery, Rothman Institute at Jefferson, Sidney Kimmel Medical College, Philadelphia, Pennsylvania, USA

AVREETA SINGH, MD
Foot and Ankle Surgery, Department of Orthopaedic Surgery, University of California, Davis, Sacramento, California, USA

JOHN R. STEELE, MD
Foot and Ankle Division, Department of Orthopedic Surgery, Duke University Medical Center, Durham, North Carolina, USA

BRIAN D. STEGINSKY, DO
Fellow, Illinois Bone & Joint Institute, Libertyville, Illinois, USA

PAUL SWITAJ, MD
OrthoVirginia, Reston, Virginia, USA

BRYAN VAN DYKE, DO
Fellow, The Orthopedic Foot & Ankle Center, Westerville, Ohio, USA

JACOB R. ZIDE, MD
Orthopaedic Surgeon, Foot and Ankle Surgery Division, Baylor University Medical Center, Clinical Professor, Texas A&M University Health Science Center, Dallas, Texas, USA

Editorial Advisory Board

Contents

Chronic Achilles tendon ruptures are debilitating injuries and are often associated with large tendon gaps that can be challenging for the foot and ankle surgeon to treat. Preoperative evaluation should include the patient's functional goals, medical comorbidities, MRI assessment of gastrocsoleus muscle viability, condition of adjacent flexor tendons, and size of the tendon defect. Although several surgical techniques have been described, the surgeon must formulate an individualized treatment plan for the patient. This article reviews the principles of diagnosis, treatment options, and clinical outcomes, and outlines the authors' preferred techniques.

Although most astute clinicians can diagnose Achilles tendon ruptures by physical examination alone, more than 20% are not accurately diagnosed in a timely fashion. The definition of a "chronic" Achilles tendon rupture in the foot and ankle literature varies widely: from 4 to 10 weeks status after injury. Neglected or chronic Achilles tendon ruptures can be significantly disabling to patients if the muscle-tendon unit is stretched beyond its normal passive limit. There are a variety of treatment options that all have valid uses but have not been proved to be superior to one another.

Noninsertional Achilles tendinosis is differentiated from insertional Achilles tendinosis based on anatomic location. Tendinosis, as opposed to tendonitis, is primarily a degenerative process, and the role of inflammation is believed limited. The etiology of Achilles tendinopathy may include overuse leading to repetitive microtrauma, poor vascularity of the tissue, mechanical imbalances of the extremity, or a combination of these elements. There is evidence to support eccentric exercise nonoperative management for patients with noninsertional Achilles tendinopathy. Operative treatment options include percutaneous longitudinal tenotomies, minimally invasive tendon scraping, open debridement and tubularization, and tendon augmentation with flexor hallucis longus.

Insertional Achilles tendinopathy is a degenerative enthesopathy associated with pain and dysfunction. Nonsurgical management is first attempted for a period of 3 to 6 months and may consist of physical therapy with eccentric training and other modalities. Surgical treatment can be successful with a variety of approaches. A thorough debridement through a midline tendon-splitting approach is associated with high satisfaction rates. Flexor hallucis longus transfer to augment the repair is considered in older, heavier patients or if more than 50% of the tendon was debrided. Early functional rehabilitation is associated with excellent outcomes.

Endoscopically assisted procedures have been established to provide the surgeon with minimally invasive techniques to address common Achilles conditions. Modifications to some of these techniques as well as improvements in instrumentation have allowed these procedures to provide similar clinical results to the traditional open surgeries while reducing wound complications and accelerating patient's recoveries. The available literature on these techniques reports consistently good outcomes with few complications, making them appealing for surgeons to adopt.

Surgical management of Achilles disorders warrants excision of the degenerated tendon and removal of impinging bone. Resulting defects can be bridged by various methods. Although flexor hallucis longus is the most commonly used tendon for transfer, large defects in cases of chronic Achilles ruptures may be bridged by use of a distant donor tendon. Bony anchorage of a lengthened or transferred tendon into the calcaneus can be done with suture anchors or with interference screws. In developing countries, such implants may not be available or affordable, necessitating the adoption of innovative ways to anchor tendons into the calcaneus.

Tibialis anterior (TA) tendon rupture is a rare injury that has been described and studied in the orthopedic literature through case reports and low-volume case studies. This article reviews the current literature on TA tendinosis and acute and chronic ruptures. It discusses the patient presentation, physical examination, nonoperative management, surgical treatment options, and outcomes.

A high clinical suspicion and greater understanding of the anatomy and pathophysiology of lateral ankle injuries have enabled early diagnosis and treatment-improving outcomes of acute peroneal tendon tears. Multiple conditions can be the cause of lateral ankle pain attributed to the peroneal tendons: tenosynovitis, tendinosis, subluxation and dislocation, stenosing tenosynovitis, abnormality related to the os peroneum, as well as tears of the peroneal tendons. It is imperative for the clinician to maintain a high suspicion for peroneal tendon abnormality when evaluating patients with lateral ankle pain.

Chronic rupture of the peroneal tendons can be a functionally limiting condition with a multitude of causes. Conservative and operative interventions
are heterogenous and tailored to the functional demands of the patient.
Surgical plans are based on muscle viability, patient preference, and surgeon expertise. Clinical outcomes evidence remains limited in this domain,
and further well-designed studies are warranted to guide treatment.

FOOT AND ANKLE CLINICS

THE CLINICS ARE NOW AVAILABLE ONLINE!
Access your subscription at:
www.theclinics.com

Preface

All Those Worms

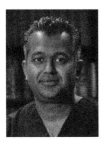

Selene G. Parekh, MD, MBA, FAOA
Editor

Dating back to the time of Homer, man has been intrigued by tendons. Achilles, the most popular and well known of the lot, has been a hot topic of debate for years. Treatment of acute to chronic issues, nonop versus surgical care, open versus percutaneous, the use of adjunctive treatments or not, and so much more have been argued. Many countries are not afforded the luxury of fancy tools that allow surgeons to help our patients. In this issue, we touch on the current state of many of these topics and have authors who discuss their implant-free methods of handling these issues in their own country.

Advances in peroneal tendon treatment have evolved as well. We have come a long way from the times of offering only repairs or tenodeses. Now we have options for allografts, tendon transfers, and the use of adjuncts as well. Fibular osteotomies can be performed in a variety of ways. Some of the authors in this issue will elucidate and expand on these treatment algorithms.

Such insight will also be given in this issue to the often neglected anterior tibial tendon. Although we don't see these abnormalities as frequently, anterior tibial tendon issues can lead to significant morbidity. The advances from both the Achilles and the peroneals can be applied to the anterior tibial tendon.

Since the time I have been in practice, I have been intrigued by tendons. Looking like worms, and even more so if they are completely torn on an MRI, these are structures on which we have struggled to provide clear guidelines for care. From the general orthopedist to the sports medicine surgeons, to the traumatologists, tendon abnormalities are diagnosed and treated by many of us. In recent years, the understanding of the basic science behind these abnormalities is expanding and it is hoped will one day allow us to intervene and treat tendinopathies long before surgery is required.

While reading this issue, you will find the latest thoughts on the process, diagnosis, and treatment of tendon abnormalities. Keep in mind that as our knowledge evolves,

Foot Ankle Clin N Am 22 (2017) xv–xvi
https://doi.org/10.1016/j.fcl.2017.09.001
1083-7515/17/© 2017 Published by Elsevier Inc.

foot.theclinics.com

so too will our treatments. In the end, it is about returning our patients to function in the most efficient manner.

Selene G. Parekh, MD, MBA, FAOA
North Carolina Orthopaedic Clinic
Department of Orthopaedic Surgery
Fuqua School of Business
Duke University
3609 SW Durham Drive
Durham, NC 27707, USA

E-mail address:
selene.parekh@gmail.com

Understanding the Anatomy and Biomechanics of Ankle Tendons

Christopher P. Chiodo, MD

KEYWORDS

- Tendon biomechanics • Tendon anatomy • Ankle tendons

KEY POINTS

- The composition and structure of tendons is complex. Molecular and biomechanical features unique to tendons allow for both strength and flexibility.
- Tendons have an ordered and hierarchical structure and comprise densely packed parallel yet staggered collagen fibrils, which results in high tensile strength.
- The tendon insertion may be either fibrous or fibrocartilaginous. The 4 zones of the latter include tendon, uncalcified fibrocartilage, calcified fibrocartilage, and bone.
- The particular anatomy of the Achilles, posterior tibial, anterior tibial, and peroneal tendons facilitates the unique function of each tendon.

INTRODUCTION

The tendons of the foot and ankle are complex and unique structures. In healthy individuals, they transmit large loads across several joints thousands of times each day. They also enable such diverse functions as standing, squatting, and running. The insertion of a tendon, which withstands several times body weight, rarely fails and might even be considered a controlled malignancy in which one tissue rigidly invades another.

This article reviews the intricate anatomy and biomechanics of the major tendon groups that cross the ankle and hindfoot, including the Achilles, anterior tibial, posterior tibial, and peroneal tendons.

TENDON COMPOSITION AND STRUCTURE

Tendons are a dense connective tissue designed to connect muscle to bone. In so doing, they transmit muscular forces across a joint and thereby produce motion.

The author has nothing to disclose.
Department of Orthopaedic Surgery, Brigham and Women's Hospital, 1153 Centre Street, Boston, MA 02181, USA
E-mail address: cchiodo@partners.org

Foot Ankle Clin N Am 22 (2017) 657–664
http://dx.doi.org/10.1016/j.fcl.2017.07.001
1083-7515/17/© 2017 Elsevier Inc. All rights reserved.

The dry weight of tendons comprises primarily type I collagen.[1] Type I collagen has superior tensile strength and, gram for gram, is reported to be stronger than steel.[2] Other proteins present in tendon include type III collagen, elastin, and fibronectin. As its name implies, elastin imparts elasticity to the tendon so that it can recoil after stretching. Meanwhile, fibronectin is a cell attachment molecule that is found on the periphery of tendons and likely facilitates gliding and lubrication.[3] Proteoglycans such as decorin and aggrecan are also present in tendon and play important roles in attracting water, lubrication, and the interconnection of tendon fibrils.[4]

At the supramolecular level, tendons have an orderly and hierarchal structure, which imparts substantial tensile strength and allows them to withstand the large forces generated by skeletal muscle contraction (**Fig. 1**). Densely packed parallel yet staggered collagen fibrils together form primary and secondary collagen fibers and bundles.[5] The tendon bundles are oriented parallel to the long axis of the tendon, which increases tensile strength. In the relaxed state, collagen bundles also have a wavelike or undulating pattern called *crimp* (**Fig. 2**). As Herchenhan and colleagues[6] note, unbuckling of the crimped collagen bundles during tenocyte contraction acts as shock absorber on initial loading and facilitates elastic recoil. Franchi and colleagues[7] also showed the presence of smaller fibrillar crimps that may act as a shock absorber during eccentric contraction.

As noted, the insertion of a tendon, or enthesis, is an impressive anatomic structure with remarkable pull-out strength. An enthesis may be either fibrous or fibrocartilaginous. Fibrous entheses are typically broad and have metaphyseal or diaphyseal insertions. These include the posterior tibial, peroneal, and tibialis anterior tendons. Meanwhile, fibrocartilaginous entheses typically occur at an epiphysis or apophysis, such as the Achilles at the calcaneal tuberosity. These entheses are characterized by a transition of tissue composition through 4 zones: tendon, uncalcified fibrocartilage, calcified fibrocartilage, and bone (**Fig. 3**). These zones allow for a more gradual transition from flexible to stiff tissue quality and also serve to dissipate stress as the tendon bends around its bony attachment point.

Fibrocartilaginous entheses may be more susceptible to overuse injury.[8] Although the midsubstance of a tendon is subject primarily to tensile loads, the tendon insertion is exposed to both compressive and tensile forces. Considering the Achilles, the anterior portion of the tendon insertion is exposed to high compressive loads as it courses over the calcaneal tuberosity. As described by Docking and colleagues,[9] tendons

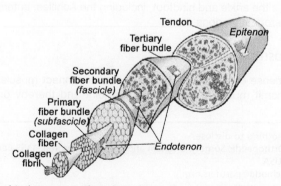

Fig. 1. The hierarchical structure of tendons. (*From* Sharma P, Maffulli N. Tendon injury and tendinopathy: healing and repair. J Bone Joint Surg Am 2005;87(1):187–202; with permission.)

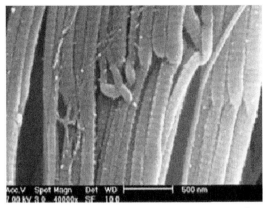

Fig. 2. Electron micrograph shows Achilles tendon crimp. (*From* Franchi M, Fini M, Quaranta M, et al. Crimp morphology in relaxed and stretched rat Achilles tendon. J Anat 2007;210(1):1–7; with permission.)

show adaptive responses when subjected to compression, including the development of fibrocartilage. With excessive or sudden increases in load, a patient may develop tendinopathy, characterized by cell proliferation and the production of disorganized collagen and extracellular matrix.[10]

Like other soft tissues in the body, tendons have both viscous and elastic properties and are therefore considered viscoelastic. With this, they exhibit time-dependent strain. The stress strain curve of tendons has been extensively investigated and has 3 major regions (**Fig. 4**). With initial load, the collagen fibrils uncrimp. This uncramping is referred to as the *toe* region of the stress strain curve and is representative of the stress created by normal, physiologic muscle contraction. Subsequently, the collagen fibers themselves are stretched and slide past one another. Without the buffer of the crimp, the collagen fibers are stiffer, and the stress strain curve becomes linear. In this linear region, the tendon exhibits elastic deformation. With increasing load, structural damage and fibril failure occur, which is the yield and failure region, and is characterized by plastic deformation with decreased stiffness and strain. The transition point between the linear and failure regions is referred to as the *elastic limit* or the *yield point*.

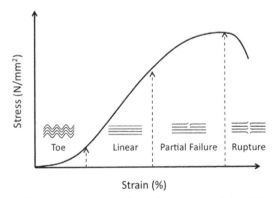

Fig. 3. Histology of a fibrocartilaginous enthesis. (*From* Apostolakos J, Durant TJ, Dwyer CR, et al. The enthesis: a review of the tendon-to-bone insertion. Muscles Ligaments Tendons J 2014;4(3):333–42; with permission.)

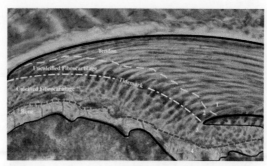

Fig. 4. Stress strain curve for normal tendon. (*From* Sharma P, Maffulli N. Tendon injury and tendinopathy: healing and repair. J Bone Joint Surg Am 2005;87(1):187–202; with permission.)

ACHILLES TENDON

In Greek mythology, Achilles was the son of Thetis, a sea nymph and the goddess of water. After his birth, Thetis dipped Achilles in the river Styx to bestow immortality. When doing so, she held him by the heel and as such this region of his body did not come in contact with the protective waters of the Styx. Later in life, Achilles would become a hero of the Trojan wars. Ultimately, however, he was killed when shot in the heel by a poison arrow. This is the origin of the phrase "Achilles heel" and the name of one of the strongest and largest tendons of the body.

The Achilles tendon connects the terminal fibers of the triceps surae, which comprises gastrocnemius and soleus muscles, to the posterior tuberosity of the calcaneus. When present, the plantaris muscle and tendon also coalesce with the Achilles. As they descend, the fibers of the Achilles internally rotate, which decreases buckling when the tendon is slack and deformation when it is loaded. It may also reduce fiber distortion and interfiber friction.[11]

Simply stating that the triceps surae and Achilles tendon are the main plantarflexors of the ankle joint is an oversimplification of the complex biomechanics of this motor unit. The soleus and gastrocnemius muscles have unique characteristics and different roles. The gastrocnemius crosses both the knee and ankle and has a higher proportion of fast twitch fibers. This configuration allows for the rapid propulsion necessary for running and jumping. On the other hand, the soleus does not cross the knee joint and has a higher proportion of slow twitch fibers when compared with the gastrocnemius. It thus serves as a postural muscle, firing when a person is standing still.

The triceps surae and Achilles can also have an eversion or inversion or moment arm, as seen with a valgus or varus hindfoot, respectively. This may result in an undesired deforming force, and is an important consideration when contemplating realignment procedures. On the other hand, such coronal moment arms may be protective. In the neutral hindfoot, the Achilles can have an inversion moment arm in eversion and an eversion one in inversion.[12] In other words, the Achilles may play a role in resisting the extremes of hindfoot motion.

ANTERIOR TIBIAL TENDON

The tibialis anterior muscle serves as the antagonist to the triceps surae and is the primary dorsiflexor of the ankle joint. Concentric contraction during the swing phase of gait allows the foot to clear the ground while eccentric contraction during early stance phase allows for controlled return of the foot to the ground.

The tibialis anterior muscle originates from the proximal two-thirds of the lateral tibia. Distally, the tibialis anterior tendon travels deep to the superior and inferior extensor retinaculum. These structures prevent bowstringing and extensor lag. The tendon inserts primarily on the first metatarsal base and medial cuneiform, medial to the sagittal midline. As such, coronal plane balance necessitates a motor unit with a corresponding dorsiflexion moment that is lateral to the midline, and this is provided by the extensor digitorum longs and peroneus tertius.

This anatomic interplay is important when it comes to treating a recurrent clubfoot or equinovarus deformity. Specifically, the vector of the unbalanced anterior tibial tendon can cause supination of the foot. In these situations the tendon must often be lateralized. Hui and colleagues[13] found that when transferring the whole tendon, it should be anchored in line with the third metatarsal. Meanwhile, when performing a split anterior tibial tendon transfer, inserting the lateral limb along the fourth metatarsal axis was most effective.

POSTERIOR TIBIAL TENDON

Although the Achilles and anterior tibial tendons allow for forward propulsion through ankle dorsiflexion and plantarflexion in the sagittal plane, coronal plane motion and stability is also necessary for ambulation on uneven terrain. This is made possible by the joints of the hindfoot, which, in turn, are stabilized by the posterior tibial and peroneal tendons.

The tibialis posterior muscle originates from the posterior tibia, fibula, and interosseus membrane. It lies in the deep posterior compartment of the leg, adjacent to the interosseus membrane and deep to the posterior tibial nerve and vessels. Distally, the posterior tibial tendon runs behind the medial malleolus and is stabilized here by the flexor retinaculum. The tendon has a broad insertion in the midfoot. The primary insertion is the navicular tuberosity. However, secondary slips also attach to the cuneiforms, cuboid, sustentaculum tali, and second through fourth metatarsal bases.

The primary function of the posterior tibial tendon is to invert the hindfoot just after heel strike during the stance phase of the gait cycle. Because the tendon travels posterior to the medial malleolus, it also plantarflexes the ankle. With inversion, the hindfoot locks and becomes a rigid lever for push-off; this happens as a result of the dynamic alignment of the axes of the subtalar and transverse tarsal joints. Specifically, these axes are parallel at heel strike. With this, the hindfoot is more flexible and serves as a shock absorber. As the foot progresses through stance, hindfoot inversion causes the axes to diverge, and the hindfoot becomes more rigid. Rather than absorbing the force of heel strike, the hindfoot now converts to a lever, making push-off and forward propulsion more efficient.

The posterior tibial tendon is also the dynamic stabilizer of the medial longitudinal arch. In this capacity, it supports and protects the calcaneonavicular or Spring ligament, which is the static stabilizer of the arch. The arches of the feet are important for several reasons, including structural support, shock absorption, and transmission of tendons and neurovascular structures.

With deficiency, dysfunction, or tearing of the posterior tibial tendon, increased load is placed on the medical longitudinal arch and talonavicular joint. Further, the eversion moment of the peroneal tendons is unopposed, which may ultimately lead to attenuation and failure of the Spring ligament, resulting in an adult acquired flatfoot deformity. Using a multisegment biomechanical model, Arangio and Salathe[14] have demonstrated that posterior tibial tendon dysfunction leads to increased load on the talonavicular joint, and that a 10-mm medial displacement calcaneal osteotomy can reduce this force back to normal values.[14]

PERONEAL TENDONS

The peroneal tendons run in a shared synovial sheath along the posterolateral ankle and hindfoot. Just distal to the fibula, they travel in separate fibro-osseous tunnels and are separated by the peroneal tubercle of the calcaneus. The primary function of the peroneals is to evert and stabilize the joints of the hindfoot. Otis and colleagues[15] found that the peroneus brevis is a more effective evertor than the peroneus longus. In addition, the peroneus longus is a strong plantarflexor of the first metatarsal.

Peroneus Brevis

The peroneus brevis muscle originates from the distal two-thirds of the lateral fibula. As it courses distally, the brevis tendon emerges as a broad and ribbon-shaped structure. At the level of the ankle, it sits immediately posterior to the fibula in the peroneal groove of this bone. Here it is stabilized by the superior peroneal retinaculum and is vulnerable to longitudinal tears that may result from instability, tendinosis, or both. Distally, the brevis tendon passes through a fibro-osseous tunnel in the hindfoot and then inserts on the base of the fifth metatarsal.

As noted, the primary role of the peroneus brevis is to evert the hindfoot. The peroneus brevis muscle contracts during mid to late stance. This stabilizes the hindfoot and also returns it to an everted and supple position in preparation for heel strike. Otis and colleagues[15] found in a cadaver model that the brevis is a more effective evertor than the longus.

The peroneals are also important dynamic stabilizers of the ankle joint. More specifically, they are integral to opposing inversion moments and protecting the tibiotalar joint from inversion injury. In this capacity, they serve to augment and protect the underlying lateral ligaments, which, along with the capsule, are the static stabilizers of the joint. To this end, Ashton-Miller and colleagues[16] found that evertor muscle strength compares favorably to taping, orthoses, and shoe height when it comes to protecting the inverted, weight-bearing ankle against further inversion.

Although mechanical lateral ligament instability may be caused by ligamentous laxity, functional ankle instability may in part be caused by peroneal tendon dysfunction. Méndez-Rebolledo and colleagues[17] recently found that the peroneals had longer reaction times and reduced postural control in basketball players with functional ankle instability. Similar findings were also reported by Donahue and colleagues.[18]

Peroneus Longus

The peroneus longus tendon has a rather circuitous route. It descends vertically with the peroneus brevis posterior to the fibula and then courses anteriorly along the lateral hindfoot. In the region of the calcaneocuboid joint, it again changes direction, coursing medially and obliquely toward the base of the first metatarsal. Here it enters a groove in the inferior aspect of the cuboid and is stabilized by the long plantar ligament. In approximately 25% of individuals an os peroneum bone is present, serving as a fulcrum and improving the tendon's efficiency.[19] After traveling across the foot, it inserts on the lateral aspect of the first metatarsal base and medial cuneiform.

Although the peroneus brevis everts the hindfoot, it also plantarflexes the first metatarsal. This process becomes especially relevant when treating a cavus foot or a forefoot-driven hindfoot varus. With these deformities, a peroneus longus to peroneus brevis transfer is an important consideration when formulating the surgical plan.

SUMMARY

The tendons that cross the ankle are complex and sophisticated structures that enable standing and forward propulsion and the ability to accommodate uneven ground. Understanding the biomechanics and local anatomy of these tendons is essential to the treatment of disorders of the foot and ankle, whether it be in formulating an appropriate physical therapy regimen or planning a reconstructive surgical procedure.

REFERENCES

1. Thorpe CT, Screen HR. Tendon structure and composition. Adv Exp Med Biol 2016;920:3–10.
2. Lodish H, Berk A, Zipursky SL, et al. Molecular cell biology. Section 22.3, Collagen: the fibrous proteins of the matrix. 4th edition. New York: W. H. Freeman; 2000. Available at: https://www.ncbi.nlm.nih.gov/books/NBK21582/.
3. Banes AJ, Link GW, Bevin AG, et al. Tendon synovial cells secrete fibronectin in vivo and in vitro. J Orthop Res 1988;6(1):73–82.
4. Raspanti M, Congiu T, Guizzardi S. Structural aspects of the extracellular matrix of the tendon: an atomic force and scanning electron microscopy study. Arch Histol Cytol 2002;65(1):37–43.
5. Sharma P, Maffulli N. Tendon injury and tendinopathy: healing and repair. J Bone Joint Surg Am 2005;87(1):187–202.
6. Herchenhan A, Kalson NS, Holmes DF, et al. Tenocyte contraction induces crimp formation in tendon-like tissue. Biomech Model Mechanobiol 2012;11(3–4):449–59.
7. Franchi M, Quaranta M, De Pasquale V, et al. Tendon crimps and peritendinous tissues responding to tensional forces. Eur J Histochem 2007;51(Suppl 1):9–14.
8. Apostolakos J, Durant TJ, Dwyer CR, et al. The enthesis: a review of the tendon-to-bone insertion. Muscles Ligaments Tendons J 2014;4(3):333–42.
9. Docking S, Samiric T, Scase E, et al. Relationship between compressive loading and ECM changes in tendons. Muscles, Ligaments Tendons J 2013;3(1):7–11.
10. Cook JL, Purdam C. Is compressive load a factor in the development of tendinopathy? Br J Sports Med 2012;46(3):163–8.
11. Ahmed IM, Lagopoulos M, McConnell P, et al. Blood supply of the Achilles tendon. J Orthop Res 1998;16:591–6.
12. Klein P, Mattys S, Rooze M. Moment arm length variations of selected muscles-sacting on talocrural and subtalar joints during movement: an in vitro study. J Biomech 1996;29(1):21–30.
13. Hui JH, Goh JC, Lee EH. Biomechanical study of tibialis anterior tendon transfer. Clin Orthop Relat Res 1998;(349):249–55.
14. Arangio GA, Salathe EP. A biomechanical analysis of posterior tibial tendon dysfunction, medial displacement calcaneal osteotomy and flexor digitorum longus transfer in adult acquired flat foot. Clin Biomech (Bristol, Avon) 2009;24(4):385–90.
15. Otis JC, Deland JT, Lee S, et al. Peroneus brevis is a more effective evertor than peroneus longus. Foot Ankle Int 2004;25(4):242–6.
16. Ashton-Miller JA, Ottaviani RA, Hutchinson C, et al. What best protects the inverted weightbearing ankle against further inversion? Evertor muscle strength compares favorably with shoe height, athletic tape, and three orthoses. Am J Sports Med 1996;24(6):800–9.
17. Méndez-Rebolledo G, Guzmán-Muñoz E, Gatica-Rojas V, et al. Longer reaction time of the fibularis longus muscle and reduced postural control in basketball

players with functional ankle instability: a pilot study. Phys Ther Sport 2015;16(3): 242–7.

18. Donahue MS, Docherty CL, Riley ZA. Decreased fibularis reflex response during inversion perturbations in FAI subjects. J Electromyogr Kinesiol 2014;24(1):84–9.

19. Peterson JJ, Bancroft LW. Os peroneal fracture with associated peroneus longus tendinopathy. AJR Am J Roentgenol 2001;177(1):257–8.

Tendonitis and Tendinopathy
What Are They and How Do They Evolve?

Andrew E. Federer, MD, John R. Steele, MD, Travis J. Dekker, MD,
Jordan L. Liles, MD, Samuel B. Adams, MD*

KEYWORDS

- Tendinopathy • Degenerative tendinopathy • Tendonitis • Achilles • Posterior tibialis
- Peroneal tendons

KEY POINTS

- The development of tendinitis and tendinopathy is often multifactorial and the result of both intrinsic and extrinsic factors.
- Intrinsic factors include anatomic factors, age-related factors, and systemic factors, whereas extrinsic factors include mechanical overload and improper form and equipment.
- Although tendinitis and tendinopathy are often incorrectly used interchangeably, they are two distinct pathologies.
- Due to their chronicity and high prevalence in tendons about the ankle, including the Achilles tendon, the posterior tibialis tendon, and the peroneal tendons, tendinitis and tendinopathies cause significant morbidity and are important pathologies for physicians to recognize.

INTRODUCTION

Tendons are dense, highly structured connective tissues that produce joint motion by transferring forces from muscle to bone. They are composed primarily of type I collagen arranged in parallel fibers, with minor constituents, such as proteoglycans, glycosaminoglycans, and other collagens constituting the remaining 20% to 30% of dry weight.[1] Although the structure and inherent characteristics of tendons give them great tensile strength and allow them to transfer force from muscle to bone, many of these same characteristics also result in poor healing potential. As such, chronic tendon problems, including tendonitis and tendinopathies, account for a significant portion of visits to primary care and sports medicine doctors. Epidemiologic studies report that work-related musculoskeletal disorders encompass more than one-third of all work days missed,

The authors have nothing to disclose.
Foot and Ankle Division, Department of Orthopedic Surgery, Duke University Medical Center, 2301 Erwin Road, Box 3000, Durham, NC 27710, USA
* Corresponding author. 4709 Creekstone Drive, Durham, NC 27703.
E-mail address: Samuel.adams@duke.edu

and the repetitive trauma disorders, such as tendinopathies, encompass more than 65% of these work-related musculoskeletal disorders.[2] Although the prevalence and incidence are variable, chronic tendon disorders comprise a significant portion of all sport-related injuries. Studies report that chronic tendon problems represent 30% of all running-related injuries and have a prevalence of almost 40% in tennis players.[3,4] These injuries are important to understand not only due to their prevalence in society but also for their chronicity in both affliction and treatment.

At their root, many chronic tendinopathies are a result of excessive mechanical load across a tendon. That is to say that the tendon was not preconditioned for the load that it is exposed to. For this reason, it is not necessarily the absolute force, duration, or frequency of load a tendon is exposed to across a period of time, but instead that these factors were in excess of the tendon's usual conditioning. The high intensity or frequency the tendon is exposed to is believed to injure the structure of the tendon. If the regenerative capabilities are not exceeded, then spontaneous healing generally occurs; however, if these capabilities are exceeded, clinical symptoms of tendinopathy occur. Inflammation is a common result, and for this reason, tendonitis is frequently the diagnosis under these circumstances. Much basic science and clinical literature, however, does not fully agree on this as the uniform reason for tendinopathies and tendonitis, and these terms are often used incorrectly.

Tendinitis is inflammation of a tendon proper, whereas tenosynovitis is inflammation of the tendon and its sheath. Tendinosis is degeneration of the collagen bundles forming the tendon tissue without significant inflammation[5] (**Table 1**). In distinguishing between these entities, it is important to understand the different types of tendons. Tendons that have altered directional courses or are bound by tunnels or retinacula often have synovial sheaths, which act to decrease the frictional forces encountered during tendon motion.[5] Tendons that are linear often do not have sheaths. With regard to commonly injured tendons of the foot and ankle, the posterior tibial tendon and peroneal tendons are sheathed tendons whereas the Achilles tendon is not. Instead, the Achilles tendon is encased with a thin, vascular layer known as the paratenon. Deep to this is a layer rich with mucopolysaccharides that allows significant freedom of movement of the Achilles.[6]

ETIOLOGY

In most cases of chronic tendon injuries, there is often a combination of intrinsic and extrinsic factors leading to injury. In many cases, a patient has an intrinsic predisposition that is subsequently exposed to an extrinsic factor, resulting in a chronic tendon injury. It has been postulated that tendinopathy in younger populations often develops in the setting of systemic inflammatory disease or secondary to trauma or intense athletics, whereas in older populations it is often the result of chronic microtrauma from overuse in the setting of age-related degeneration.[5]

Extrinsic Factors

Mechanical overload is generally considered to be one of primary causes of chronic tendinopathy. It can be further broken down into subcategories, such as increased duration, frequency, and intensity as well as errors in technique. In general, tendons respond more favorably to cyclic loading rather than large magnitudes of load.[7] A study by Simonsen and colleagues[8] showed that the Achilles tendon of rats did not strengthen with an exercise regime of high force and few cycles but that the tendons did increase in strength with endurance swimming training. Increases in tendon strength and stiffness have not been found due to hypertrophy or increases in collagen concentration, as might be suspected.

Table 1 Tendinosis versus tendinitis		
Pathology	**Histologic Changes**	**Graphic**
Tendinosis	Intratendinous degeneration of collagen fibers	
Tendinitis	Inflammation of tendon proper	

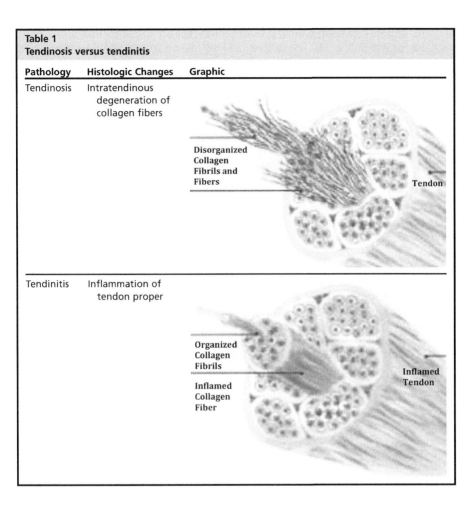

In their study of the effects of exercise on tendons, Buchanan and colleagues[7] postulated that the increased stiffness is likely a protective mechanism to reduce tendon damage by allowing less extension of the tendon under the same load. In the setting of repetitive load, however, such as long distance running that does not allow for full repair or a large magnitude load that causes macrotrauma, the tendon cannot respond in this fashion, leading to mechanical failure and tendinopathy.

Mechanical overload is often adversely supplemented by other extrinsic factors, such as improper form, inappropriate equipment from running shoes to occupational tools, and lack of protective gear. Although there is a paucity of data commenting on the extrinsic factors contributing to tendonitis, modification of these factors is often the first objective in treatment. Decreased duration, frequency, and intensity can frequently lessen the symptoms of chronic tendinopathies when discovered in its early stages (see **Table 1**).

Intrinsic Factors

Intrinsic factors that predispose someone for the development of chronic tendinopathies consist of anatomic factors, age-related factors, and systemic factors.[9]

Anatomic factors include malalignment, inflexibility, eccentric muscle use, and muscle weakness or imbalance. This, in conjunction with mechanical overload tendencies, is often implicated in chronic tendinopathies in younger patients. Age-related factors contributing to chronic tendinopathies include tendon degeneration, decreased healing response, increased tendon stiffness, and decreased vascularity. Systemic factors include diabetes mellitus, obesity, smoking, and inflammatory enthesopathies (**Fig. 1**).

Tendons receive their vascular supply through the musculotendinous junction, the osseotendinous junction, and additional supply depending on the tendon type. Sheathed tendons receive blood supply from the mesotenon and vincula, whereas tendons that are not sheathed receive blood supply from the surrounding paratenon. In general, vascularity is poor at watershed zones that exist within many tendons and it can also be compromised at sites of friction, torsion, or compression.[10] Because hypovascular zones may limit the normal inflammatory cascade and diminish the healing response, the tendon is at risk for cumulative degeneration in these areas.[10] Several studies using ultrasound in vivo have also shown that tendon vascularity decreases with age, contributing to a decreased healing response with increasing age.[11,12]

The relationship between aging and changes in the biochemical properties of tendons is unclear based on the conflicting current literature at this time. For example, some research shows that tendons increase in stiffness with age, whereas other shows that tendons increase in compliance with age.[13,14] What is not debated, however, is that as tendons age they have decreased resilience and decreased inherent healing potential. Zhou and colleagues[15] showed progenitor stem cells are reduced in number and capacity to proliferate with increasing age. These changes leave tendons less able to adapt and respond to the mechanical loads and stresses applied to them. This also lends credence to the thought process behind treatments involving platelet-rich plasma and mesenchymal stem cells, namely to stimulate the body's biologic response to healing that decreases with age. In addition, other studies have shown changes in tenocytes with age, namely decreased protein synthesis and decreased ability to repair the tendon to bone interface with age.[16,17]

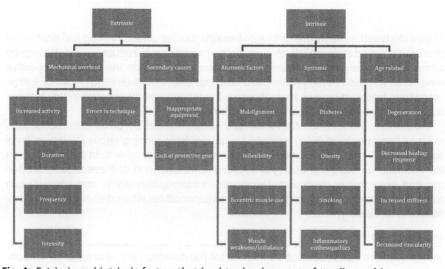

Fig. 1. Extrinsic and intrinsic factors that lead to development of tendinopathies.

Systemic factors that may contribute to the development of tendinopathy include diabetes mellitus, obesity, smoking, and inflammatory enthesopathies. Many studies have shown an association between tendinopathy and diabetes mellitus. One systematic review with meta-analysis of 31 studies by Ranger and colleagues[18] found that tendinopathy was more prevalent in people with diabetes than those without diabetes, with an odds ratio of 3.67 and a 95% CI of 2.71 to 4.97. Oliveira and colleagues[19] studied MRI changes, nanostructural changes, and inflammatory markers in tendons of rats with experimental diabetes compared with tendons of rats without diabetes. Compared with the tendon in rats without diabetes, this group found a statistically significant increase in the size of the tendons in rats with diabetes, found that the tendons of the diabetic group had greater irregularity in their fiber bundles, and found no changes in the level of inflammatory markers interleukin-1 and tumor necrosis factor α between the 2 groups. They thus concluded that diabetes mellitus promotes structural changes in tendons without major inflammatory changes. Obesity has been shown to exert harmful effects on tendons, with a multifactorial etiology consisting of mechanical overload due to increased body weight as well as increased systemic bioactive peptides, such as leptin that contribute to a chronic, low-grade inflammatory state.[20] Smoking, with its well-documented negative influences on wound healing, may inhibit tendons' ability to heal in the face of repetitive microtrauma, leading to chronic tendinopathy. Lundgreen and colleagues[21] corroborated this in their study comparing tendon histopathology in rotator cuff tears in smokers versus nonsmokers. They found that torn tendons in smokers have advanced degenerative changes, increased density of apoptotic cells, and decreased density of tenocytes compared with the torn tendons of nonsmokers, suggesting decreased tendon healing capacity in smokers. Numerous observational studies have cited an increase in tendon ruptures soon after use of fluoroquinolones. The pathoetiology is multifactorial but likely includes an up-regulation of matrix metalloproteinases (MMPs) with resulting degradation of type I collagen.[22] Systematic reviews have shown that increasing age and concomitant systemic corticosteroid use increase the likelihood of adverse events.[23,24]

PATHOLOGY: EVOLUTION

Tendons repair in response to mechanical stresses through a predictable 3-stage cycle. First, there is an inflammatory stage lasting approximately 2 days. In this stage a clot forms, bringing platelets to the area, and an inflammatory response consisting of predominately macrophages, neutrophils, growth factors, matrix MMPs, and cytokines. The next stage is a proliferation period of approximately 6 weeks where tenocytes, fibroblasts, and stem cells produce a highly cellular but weak scar that has a high percentage of type III collagen and is more randomly organized than mature tendon. Lastly, in the remodeling phase that can last up to 1 year to 2 years, the scar is replaced by normal tendon with a decrease in cellularity, an increase in type I collagen, increased longitudinal organization, and increased strength. This is the response to cyclic loading of a tendon in a suitable environment, which allows the tendon the opportunity to progress through each cycle of repair. With repetitive loading or injury, however, or in the setting of disadvantageous systemic factors, the tendon does not have the time or ability to heal itself through this normal process. Only an incomplete healing response occurs and chronic tendinopathy is often the end result.

By understanding the process of normal tendon healing, the pathology that occurs in chronic tendinopathy due to incomplete repair can be grasped. First, tendinopathy often occurs in the relative hypovascular areas of different tendons because this area may be unable to form clot and mount an effective inflammatory response. Many studies have also shown neovascularization at the site of tendinopathy, which may be the result of the tendon attempting to create a more favorable healing environment. The capillary proliferation and abnormal thick-walled vessels at these sites may, however, contribute to the symptoms of tendinopathy rather than help the problem.[25] As the inflammatory phase lingers, chronic inflammation becomes less dependent on macrophages and neutrophils although there is an up-regulation of MMPs, cytokines, painful neurotransmitters, such as substance P. Numerous studies have shown an increase in MMPs in the setting of chronic tendinopathy as well as tendon rupture.[26–28] MMPs are proteinases that degrade extracellular matrix and collagen and in the setting of tendinopathy have been shown to reduce the tensile modulus and tensile strength of tendons.[29] As the degenerative process continues, the tendon is unable to remodel the scar that was formed during the proliferative phase. This results in more the presence of more type III collagen than normal, which is weaker than type I collagen, and more random organization and irregular crosslinks of the collagen, which are not favorable for strength.

SPECIFIC TENDONS OF THE FOOT AND ANKLE
Achilles

Tendinopathies of the Achilles generally present in 1 of 3 ways: insertional tendinopathy, midsubstance tendinosis, and peritendinitis. Insertional tendinopathy is a degenerative process resulting in disorganized collagen and mucoid degeneration without a significant inflammatory component. Midsubstance tendinosis involves tendon thickening and is thought to be due to a decreased healing response to microtears of the tendon in its hypovascular zone 2 cm to 6 cm proximal to its insertion. Peritendinitis is also thought to be due to aberrant healing in the same hypovascular zone but involves inflammation of the paratenon surrounding the tendon rather than the tendon itself. The first 2 result in focal pain with tenderness to palpation whereas the third often involves more diffuse swelling around the tendon with crepitus.

Epidemiologic studies have evaluated Achilles tendinopathy in different demographics. In a cross-sectional study from the Netherlands, midportion Achilles tendinopathy seen by general practitioners accounted for 2.35 of every 1000 adult patients (21–60 years).[30] In a study evaluating nonathletes and their hindfoot angles, Achilles tendinopathy was seen in 5.6% of the 1394 feet/697 patients (4% insertional, 3.6% noninsertional, and 1.9% both). There was a 0.76° and 0.96° varus tibiocalcaneal alignment in the nonsertional and insertional tendinopathy groups, respectively, with an average valgus alignment of 1.77° for the control group.[31]

The cause of Achilles tendinopathy and tendinitis is most likely multifactorial, although some studies suggest that most painful Achilles tendinopathies demonstrate neovascularization.[32–35] Ultrasound has become a useful tool in assessing Achilles tendinopathy because it can assess tendon degeneration, as seen by hypoechoic regions, as well as tendon thickness and vascularization.[35–37] Studies conducted by the same investigators[35,37] report that in older patients who have sclerosis of the peritendinous vessels, there is less associated pain with midtendinous and insertional enthesopathic conditions. A study by van Snellenberg and colleagues,[38] however, determined that when evaluating young athletes of various sports, neovascularization (as determined by visualizing vascularization into the tendon) was only seen in 2 of 11 Achilles tendons with clinical signs of tendinopathy on examination. A total of 64 athletes and 128 tendons were evaluated and none had structural changes to the tendons.

There have been several studies commenting on the neovascularization of Achilles tendons in the presence of clinical symptoms. Although 2 studies by Ohberg and Alfredson[33,34] had shown a perfect correlation between those with chronic Achilles tendon pain having neovascularization and those patients without pain not having neovascularization, most studies have showed less definite correlations. In a case series study, Zanetti and colleagues[39] determined that 30 of 55 symptomatic tendons had neovascularization and found one of 25 contralateral asysmptomatic tendons with neovascularization. Peers and colleagues[40] found neovascularization in 22 of 25 of symptomatic tendons. Although there was no correlation with severity of pain and neovascularization, there was an association between amount of tendon degeneration and neovascularization. Several studies have reported on the existence of a prodromal period of symptoms, such as decreased plantarflexion power and pain in the Achilles tendon in a majority of elite athletes who suffered an Achilles tendon rupture.[41,42] Whether these prodromal symptoms are due to neovascularization, inflammation, or other causes is unknown at this time, but the presence of prodromal symptoms represents an opportunity for intervention prior to a potential tendon rupture.

Posterior Tibialis

The site of principal involvement of posterior tibial tendinopathy is often midsubstance as the tendon courses posterior to the medial malleolus. This is often the main component of adult acquired flatfoot deformity.[43] Posterior tibialis tendon (PTT) dysfunction is multifactorial and likely due to overuse and overload in the setting of hypovascularity; systemic factors, such as obesity; and inflammatory disorders, such as rheumatoid arthritis.[5] It is a common condition, which may have a prevalence of up to 10% in middle-aged to elderly women.[44]

There are 2 major anatomic features of the PTT that predispose it to the development of tendinopathy. First, it has a retromalleolar hypovascular region, which exists on average in the area 2.2 cm to 0.6 cm proximal to the medial malleolus based on a cadaveric study of 60 lower extremities.[45] Second, the tendon changes from a vertical to horizontal position as it courses posterior to the medial malleolus in the tarsal tunnel. This significant change of direction exposes the tendon to large frictional forces in this area. In addition, the tendon is held in position posterior to the medial malleolus by the flexor retinaculum and can be constricted by these structures, further contributing to diminished vascularity. Mechanical malalignment, excessive pronation and muscular imbalances are other anatomic abnormalities that can be present and predispose patients to PTT dysfunction.

The pathophysiology of PTT tendinopathy is often multifactorial in nature but likely due to chronic microtrauma secondary to overuse in the setting of poor intrinsic anatomic factors (discussed previously). In stage 1 of PTT dysfunction, there is tenosynovitis without deformity. Patients may complain of medial foot and ankle pain, and they are tender to palpation over the tendon.[5] As tenosynovitis lingers, chronic inflammation and synovial thickening lead to the production of granulation tissue and the degeneration of the normal collagen framework of the tendon. As the tendon degenerates over time, it weakens and fatigues under normal workloads, resulting in tears in the region of hypovascularity and friction.[46] The tendon becomes more nonfunctional and lengthens over time, and this posterior tibial tendon dysfunction leads to hindfoot valgus and pes planus deformities. The staging of PTT dysfunction is beyond the scope of this article, but, as discussed previously, there is a progressive change in peroneal tendon pathology as PTTD develops over time.[47] Although the authors are unaware of any studies documenting PTTD progression, clinical experience is that if left untreated, the pathology can progress months.

Peroneal Tendons

Peroneal tendon pathology is common and consists of tendinosis, tenosynovitis, tendon subluxation or dislocation, and tears, all of which are clinically similar in presentation. In 1 study of patients undergoing surgery for chronic lateral ankle instability, 77% had peroneal tenosynovitis, 54% had an attenuated peroneal retinaculum and 25% had a peroneus brevis tear.[48] The etiology of these pathologies are multifactorial and include prior trauma as well as mechanical overload in the setting of anatomic abnormalities or systemic factors putting the tendons at risk.

Peroneal tendinosis is a noninflammatory degeneration of the peroneal tendons that is multifactorial in nature and often seen in athletes that place repetitive stress on the lateral ankle tendons, elderly individuals, patients who have experienced ankle trauma, and those with systemic disorders, such as diabetes and inflammatory arthritis.[49] Peroneal tenosynovitis involves inflammation of the tendons or tendon sheaths and can be secondary to trauma, repetitive loads, systemic arthropathies, and infection.[50] Irregularly thickened synovium as well as synovial effusions can be seen on ultrasound with tenosynovitis, whereas MRI reveals fluid and increased signal within the tendon sheath.[50] Stenosing tenosynovitis occurs when the resulting synovial proliferation produces fibrotic tissue about the sheath or a thickened retinaculum that prevents free excursion of the peroneal tendons through their osseofibrous tunnel.[51]

Tears in the peroneus brevis and longus are also common and can be the result of acute trauma, which are not discussed in this article, or can be degenerative in nature. A shallow retromalleolar groove may contribute to tendon subluxation and subsequent tendon disorders including tearing.[52] In a retrospective review of patients treated operatively for peroneal tendon tears, 10% of patients were found to have an insufficiency of the retromalleolar groove and 20% were found to have peroneal tendon subluxation.[53] Tendinosis and tenosynovitis can weaken tendons and predispose them to degenerative tears if left untreated. In addition, tears in the peroneus longus and brevis tendons can result in irritation with continued mechanical load. The resulting chronic inflammation can thus contribute to the development of tenosynovitis.

The anatomy of the peroneal tendons also puts them at risk for the development of tendinosis and tenosynovitis. The peroneal tendons share a common synovial sheath starting 2.5 cm to 3.5 cm proximal to the tip of the fibula and develop into separate sheaths at the level of the peroneal tubercle.[54] Normally the peroneus longus is posterior to the peroneus brevis in the peroneal groove but with intrasheath subluxation these tendons can switch positions due to snapping over one another or the peroneus longus subluxating through a longitudinal tear in the peroneus brevis.[55] The superficial peroneal retinaculum acts as the main stabilizer of the peroneal tendons to maintain their position in the retromalleolar groove, but the inferior peroneal retinaculum, calcaneofibular ligament, and a fibrocartilaginous ridge along the posterolateral border of the distal fibula also work to this end. These structures can cause friction in the peroneal tendons, which can contribute to the development of tenosynovitis. In addition, the retinacula are involved in stenosing tenosynovitis, as they prevent normal excursion in the setting of hypertrophied tendon or tendon sheath. Lastly, many studies have reported that both tendons have a hypovascular zone as they wrap around the tip of the fibula, and this is commonly a location of tendon pathology.[54]

Furthermore, there are several anatomic pathologies and variants that place the peroneal tendons at risk for developing tendinitis and tendinopathy. Cavovarus deformity can contribute to tendinosis and tenosynovitis by putting the peroneal tendons at a mechanical disadvantage and causing them to be overworked. The presence of a peroneal tubercle, which is a bony protuberance off of the lateral calcaneus that is present in 40% of individuals and separates the peroneus longus and brevis tendons, can predispose the peroneus longus tendon to tenosynovitis and rupture.[56] Similarly, the presence of a peroneus quartus accessory muscle, which has a prevalence of 12% to 22%, and a low-lying peroneus brevis muscle belly can both lead to tenosynovitis, tearing, and subluxation of the peroneus brevis tendon.[57,58]

SUMMARY

The development of tendinitis and tendinopathy is often multifactorial and the result of both intrinsic and extrinsic factors. Intrinsic factors include anatomic factors, age-related factors, and systemic factors, whereas extrinsic factors include mechanical overload and improper form and equipment. Although tendinitis and tendinopathy are often incorrectly used interchangeably, they are 2 distinct pathologies. Due to their chronicity and high prevalence in tendons about the ankle, including the Achilles tendon, the PTT, and the peroneal tendons, tendinitis and tendinopathies cause significant morbidity and are important pathologies for physicians to recognize.

REFERENCES

1. Woo SL, Lee TQ, Abramowitch SD, et al. Structure and function of ligaments and tendons. In: Mow VC, Huiskes R, editors. Basic Orthopaedic Biomechanics and Mechano-biology. Philadelphia: Lippincott, Williams & Wilkins; 2005. p. 301–42.
2. Barr AE, Barbe MF, Clark BD. Work-related musculoskeletal disorders of the hand and wrist: epidemiology, pathophysiology, and sensorimotor changes. J Orthop Sports Phys Ther 2004;34(10):610–27.
3. Gruchow HW, Pelletier D. An epidemiologic study of tennis elbow. Incidence, recurrence, and effectiveness of prevention strategies. Am J Sports Med 1979; 7(4):234–8.
4. James SL, Bates BT, Osternig LR. Injuries to runners. Am J Sports Med 1978;6(2): 40–50.
5. Bare AA, Haddad SL. Tenosynovitis of the posterior tibial tendon. Foot Ankle Clin 2001;6(1):37–66.
6. Kvist M. Achilles tendon injuries in athletes. Sports Med 1994;18(3):173–201.
7. Buchanan CI, Marsh RL. Effects of exercise on the biomechanical, biochemical and structural properties of tendons. Comp Biochem Physiol A Mol Integr Physiol 2002;133(4):1101–7.
8. Simonsen EB, Klitgaard H, Bojsen-Moller F. The influence of strength training, swim training and ageing on the Achilles tendon and m. soleus of the rat. J Sports Sci 1995;13(4):291–5.
9. Almekinders LC. Tendinitis and other chronic tendinopathies. J Am Acad Orthop Surg 1998;6(3):157–64.
10. McCarthy MM, Hannafin JA. The mature athlete: aging tendon and ligament. Sports Health 2014;6(1):41–8.
11. Adler RS, Fealy S, Rudzki JR, et al. Rotator cuff in asymptomatic volunteers: contrast-enhanced US depiction of intratendinous and peritendinous vascularity. Radiology 2008;248:954–61.
12. Funakoshi T, Iwasaki N, Kamishima T, et al. In vivo visualization of vascular patterns of rotator cuff tears using contrast-enhanced ultrasound. Am J Sports Med 2010;38:2464–71.
13. Narici MV, Maffulli N, Maganaris CN. Ageing of human muscles and tendons. Disabil Rehabil 2008;30(20–22):1548–54.

14. Plate JF, Wiggins WF, Haubruck P, et al. Normal aging alters in vivo passive biomechanical response of the rat gastrocnemius-Achilles muscle-tendon unit. J Biomech 2013;46:450–5.

15. Zhou Z, Akinbiyi T, Xu L, et al. Tendon-derived stem/progenitor cell aging: defective self-renewal and altered fate. Aging Cell 2010;9:911–5.

16. Ippolito E, Natali PG, Postacchini F, et al. Morphological, immunochemical, and biochemical study of rabbit Achilles tendon at various ages. J Bone Joint Surg Am 1980;62:583–98.

17. Rodeo SA, Potter HG, Kawamura S, et al. Biologic augmentation of rotator cuff tendon-healing with use of a mixture of osteoinductive growth factors. J Bone Joint Surg Am 2007;89:2485–97.

18. Ranger TA, Wong AM, Cook JL, et al. Is there an association between tendinopathy and diabetes mellitus? A systematic review with meta-analysis. Br J Sports Med 2016;50(16):982–9.

19. Oliveira RR, Medina de Mattos R, Magalhães Rebelo L, et al. Experimental diabetes alters the morphology and nano-structure of the Achilles tendon. PLoS One 2017;12(1):e0169513.

20. Ackermann PW, Hart DA. General overview and summary of concepts regarding tendon disease topics addressed related to metabolic disorders. Adv Exp Med Biol 2016;920:293–8.

21. Lundgreen K, Lian OB, Scott A, et al. Rotator cuff tear degeneration and cell apoptosis in smokers versus nonsmokers. Arthroscopy 2014;30(8):936–41.

22. Tsai WC, Hsu CC, Chen CP, et al. Ciprofloxacin up-regulates tendon cells to express matrix metalloproteinase-2 with degradation of type I collagen. J Orthop Res 2011;29(1):67–73.

23. Hall MM, Finnoff JT, Smith J. Musculoskeletal complications of fluoroquinolones: guidelines and precautions for usage in the athletic population. PM R 2011;3(2): 132–42.

24. Stephenson AL, Wu W, Cortes D, et al. Tendon injury and fluoroquinolone use: a systematic review. Drug Saf 2013;36(9):709–21.

25. Yang X, Coleman DP, Pugh ND, et al. The volume of the neovascularity and its clinical implications in Achilles tendinopathy. Ultrasound Med Biol 2012;38: 1887–95.

26. Godoy-Santos AL, Trevisan R, Fernandes TD, et al. Association of MMP-8 polymorphisms with tendinopathy of the primary posterior tibial tendon: a pilot study. Clinics (Sao Paulo) 2011;66(9):1641–3.

27. Järvinen M, Józsa L, Kannus P, et al. Histopathological findings in chronic tendon disorders. Scand J Med Sci Sports 1997;7:86–95.

28. Kannus P, Józsa L. Histopathological changes preceding spontaneous rupture of a tendon. A controlled study of 891 patients. J Bone Joint Surg Am 1991;73: 1507–25.

29. Lavagnino M, Arnoczky SP. In vitro alterations in cytoskeletal tensional homeostasis control gene expression in tendon cells. J Orthop Res 2005;23:1211–8.

30. de Jonge S, van den Berg C, de Vos RJ, et al. Incidence of midportion Achilles tendinopathy in the general population. Br J Sports Med 2011;45(13):1026–8.

31. Waldecker U, Hofmann G, Drewitz S. Epidemiologic investigation of 1394 feet: coincidence of hindfoot malalignment and Achilles tendon disorders. Foot Ankle Surg 2012;18(2):119–23.

32. Alfredson H, Ohberg L, Forsgren S. Is vasculo-neural ingrowth the cause of pain in chronic achilles tendinosis? An investigation using ultrasonography and colour

Doppler, immunohistochemistry, and diagnostic injections. Knee Surg Sports Traumatol Arthrosc 2003;11(5):334–8.

33. Ohberg L, Alfredson H. Ultrasound guided sclerosis of neovessels in painful chronic Achilles tendinosis: pilot study of a new treatment. Br J Sports Med 2002;36(3):173–5 [discussion: 176–7].

34. Ohberg L, Alfredson H. Sclerosing therapy in chronic Achilles tendon insertional pain-results of a pilot study. Knee Surg Sports Traumatol Arthrosc 2003;11(5): 339–43.

35. Ohberg L, Lorentzon R, Alfredson H. Neovascularisation in Achilles tendons with painful tendinosis but not in normal tendons: an ultrasonographic investigation. Knee Surg Sports Traumatol Arthrosc 2001;9(4):233–8.

36. Fornage BD. Achilles tendon: US examination. Radiology 1986;159(3):759–64.

37. Ohberg L, Lorentzon R, Alfredson H. Eccentric training in patients with chronic Achilles tendinosis: normalised tendon structure and decreased thickness at follow up. Br J Sports Med 2004;38(1):8–11 [discussion: 11].

38. van Snellenberg W, Wiley JP, Brunet G. Achilles tendon pain intensity and level of neovascularization in athletes as determined by color Doppler ultrasound. Scand J Med Sci Sports 2007;17(5):530–4.

39. Zanetti M, Metzdorf A, Kundert HP, et al. Achilles tendons: clinical relevance of neovascularization diagnosed with power Doppler US. Radiology 2003;227(2): 556–60.

40. Peers KH, Brys PP, Lysens RJ. Correlation between power Doppler ultrasonography and clinical severity in Achilles tendinopathy. Int Orthop 2003;27(3):180–3.

41. Maffulli N, Longo UG, Maffulli GD, et al. Achilles tendon ruptures in elite athletes. Foot Ankle Int 2011;32(1):9–15.

42. Parekh SG, Wray WH 3rd, Brimmo O, et al. Epidemiology and outcomes of Achilles tendon ruptures in the national football league. Foot Ankle Spec 2009;2(6): 283–6.

43. Gluck GS, Heckman DS, Parekh SG. Tendon disorders of the foot and ankle, part 3: the posterior tibial tendon. Am J Sports Med 2010;38(10):2133–44.

44. Kohls-Gatzoulis J, Angel J, Singh D. Tibialis posterior dysfunction as a cause of flatfeet in elderly patients. Foot Ankle Clin 2004;14:207–9.

45. Manske MC, McKeon KE, Johnson JE, et al. Arterial anatomy of the tibialis posterior tendon. Foot Ankle Int 2015;36(4):436–43.

46. Blake RL, Anderson K, Ferguson H. Posterior tibial tendinitis. J Am Podiatr Med Assoc 1994;84:141–9.

47. Johnson KA, Strom DE. Tibialis posterior tendon dysfunction. Clin Orthop Relat Res 1989;239:196–206.

48. DiGiovanni BF, Fraga CJ, Cohen BE, et al. Associated injuries found in chronic lateral ankle instability. Foot Ankle Int 2000;21(10):809–15.

49. Roster B, Michelier P, Giza E. Peroneal tendon disorders. Clin Sports Med 2015; 34(4):625–41.

50. Lee SJ, Jacobson JA, Kim SM, et al. Ultrasound and MRI of the peroneal tendons and associated pathology. Skeletal Radiol 2013;42(9):1191–200.

51. Vuillemin V, Guerini H, Bard H, et al. Stenosing tenosynovitis. J Ultrasound 2012; 15(1):20–8.

52. Heckman DS, Reddy S, Pedowitz D, et al. Operative treatment for peroneal tendon disorders. J Bone Joint Surg Am 2008;90:404–18.

53. Dombek MF, Lamm BM, Saltrick K, et al. Peroneal tendon tears: a retrospective review. J Foot Ankle Surg 2003;42:250–8.

54. Altchek DW, DiGiovanni CW, Dines JS, et al. Foot and ankle sports medicine. Philadelphia: LippinCott Williams & Wilkins; 2013.

55. Raikin SM, Elias I, Nazarian LN. Intrasheath subluxation of the peroneal tendons. J Bone Joint Surg Am 2008;90(5):992–9.

56. Bruce WD, Christofersen MR, Phillips DL. Stenosing tenosynovitis and impingement of the peroneal tendons associated with hypertrophy of the peroneal tubercle. Foot Ankle Int 1999;20(7):464–7.

57. Sobel M, Pavlov H, Geppert MJ, et al. Painful os peroneum syndrome: a spectrum of conditions responsible for plantar lateral foot pain. Foot Ankle Int 1994; 15(3):112–24.

58. Wang XT, Rosenberg ZS, Mechlin MB, et al. Normal variants and diseases of the peroneal tendons and superior peroneal retinaculum: MR imaging features. Radiographics 2005;25(3):587–602.

Presentation, Diagnosis, and Nonsurgical Treatment Options of the Anterior Tibial Tendon, Posterior Tibial Tendon, Peroneals, and Achilles

Ⓡ CrossMark

David Pedowitz, MS, MD*, David Beck, MD

KEYWORDS

- Anterior tibial tendon • Achilles • Peroneals • Posterior tibial tendon

KEY POINTS

- Disorders of the anterior tibial tendon (ATT) are rare, and relatively few series have been described in the literature.
- Ruptures of the ATT are more common than tendinopathies of the ATT.
- For those patients with a tendinopathy, initial treatment may include activity and shoe-wear modifications.

INTRODUCTION

Disorders of the tendons of the foot and ankle are common and frequently drive patients to seek orthopedic evaluation. Many of these disorders may be treated effectively with nonsurgical options. However, it is important that one has a thorough understanding of both the presentation and the diagnosis of these disorders as well as the nonsurgical treatment options. Please see Oliver Schipper and Bruce Cohen's article, "The Acute Injury of the Achilles: Surgical Options (Open Treatment, and, Minimally Invasive Surgery)," in this issue for further discussion on disorders of the anterior tibial, posterior tibial, peroneal, and Achilles tendons.

ANTERIOR TIBIAL TENDON

Disorders of the anterior tibial tendon (ATT) are rare, and relatively few series have been described in the literature. The most common abnormalities of the ATT are

The authors have nothing to disclose.
The Rothman Institute, 825 Old Lancaster Road, Suite 202, Bryn Mawr, PA 19010, USA
* Corresponding author.
E-mail address: drpedowitz@yahoo.com

Foot Ankle Clin N Am 22 (2017) 677–687
http://dx.doi.org/10.1016/j.fcl.2017.07.012
1083-7515/17/© 2017 Elsevier Inc. All rights reserved.

foot.theclinics.com

lacerations and closed ruptures, although tendinopathies have also been described.[1–9] Although most surgeons who dedicate their practice to the treatment of foot and ankle disorders encounter ATT ruptures a few times a year, their documentation in the literature is scant. Anagnostakos and colleagues[1] performed the most extensive review of the literature and found only 110 cases of ATT rupture documented. Nonetheless, because this abnormality is relatively uncommon, recognition and diagnosis are important to prevent a missed opportunity for early treatment.

HISTORY AND PRESENTATION

Ruptures of the ATT are more common than tendinopathies of the ATT. Ruptures can be secondary to open direct trauma, closed indirect trauma, or can be spontaneous.[1] Spontaneous ruptures typically occur in older patients, particularly men between the ages of 50 and 70. Although the ruptures can occur secondary to a degenerative process, there are rarely prodromal symptoms before disruption to alert the patient or physician to impending rupture. Spontaneous ruptures are known to occur in patients with gout, inflammatory arthritis, diabetes, or steroid injections.[1,7,10–12] Corticosteroid injections into a symptomatic tendon or at its insertion are also thought to precipitate rupture when preexisting abnormality exists.

As the ATT is the primary dorsiflexor of the ankle, as well as an invertor of the foot, the mechanism of injury is typically a forceful plantarflexion to a contracted ATT. In the acute setting, patients are more likely to present with swelling and pain associated with the rupture. In chronic ruptures, patients are less likely to recall a traumatic event and may not complain of pain, but rather difficulty with gait. Specifically, they may complain of the inability to clear their toes from the ground especially on uneven ground, which can lead to tripping and falling.[1,8]

Tendinopathy is a less frequent abnormality of the ATT, but has been described in the literature as well.[3,4] Beischer and colleagues[3] reviewed a series of mostly middle-aged women who complained of swelling and pain over the ATT insertion, which was more bothersome at night. Insertional tendinopathy was also described, but typically occurred as an overuse injury.

DIAGNOSIS
Clinical Examination

On walking into the examination room, the patient's gait should be observed and may exhibit a foot drop or steppage gait. However, much of the dorsiflexion is compensated by the Extensor Hallucis Longus/Extensor Digitorum Longus and may allow dorsiflexion to neutralize.[1] Signs of toe extensor recruitment for dorsiflexion should be observed during gait.[3] An attempt to heel walk may demonstrate that the patient is unable to do so on the affected side. The ATT may retract to the level of the ankle joint leading to a visible prominence at this level (PIC).

Physical examination can reveal swelling and pain anteriorly, although these findings may be absent in a chronic injury.[9] Inspection and palpation may reveal the lack of normal contour of the anterior ankle in dorsiflexion and the absence of a palpable tendon. In addition, the patient may have difficulty dorsiflexing and inverting the foot. Typically, the foot will evert with attempted dorsiflexion. Motor strength testing may reveal weakness in dorsiflexion when compared with the uninjured leg.

Tendinopathy of the ATT may have more subtle clinical findings. Beischer and colleagues[3] described that point tenderness is maximal at the insertion of the ATT, and pain can be elicited with ankle plantarflexion, hindfoot eversion, midfoot abduction, and pronation. Force is applied to the foot in an attempt to passively stretch the TA tendon. A thorough neurologic examination should be performed because this condition can mimic a peroneal palsy or L4-5 radiculopathy.

Imaging Studies

Radiographs should be obtained to rule out other causes of pain and to evaluate underlying abnormalities that could lead to ATT disruption (gout, exostoses, tibial fracture). Ultrasound has been used to diagnose ATT ruptures as well as tendinopathies. Ultrasound can show signs of rupture, including disorganization of tendon fibers, edema, and anechoic zone corresponding to the rupture site.[13] It has also been used to diagnose tendinopathies. MRI is the mainstay of imagining modalities for evaluating abnormality of tendons. MRI will clearly demonstrate local edema, thickening of the tendon, tears or ruptures in the tendon, and reactive bone edema in the setting of insertional tendinopathy.[14,15]

NONSURGICAL TREATMENT OPTIONS

Both nonsurgical and surgical treatment options have been described and effectively used for the treatment of ATT disorders.[1,3,4,6] For those patients with a tendinopathy, initial treatment may include activity and shoe-wear modifications. A trial of bracing, CAM boot, or ankle-foot orthosis (AFO) may be attempted to alleviate symptoms before surgical intervention.[4] Steroid injections have been associated with tendon ruptures and should be avoided in this context.[10] It is generally agreed upon that complete ruptures of the ATT should be treated surgically, although there is a paucity of literature on the topic. In a young patient with acute rupture, surgical intervention is certainly indicated. In the authors' experience, except in the instance of an acute laceration, direct repair is not possible, and reconstruction using a tendon graft may be required. In elderly patients with chronic injuries and lower demand, there is more of an argument to be made for nonsurgical treatment.[1,4,6] In these cases, a trial of bracing or AFO may be attempted. In elderly patients, Markarian and colleagues[6] demonstrated effective nonsurgical treatment of ATT ruptures that led to acceptable foot and ankle function in this population.

POSTERIOR TIBIAL TENDON

Posterior tibial tendon (PTT) dysfunction is the most common acquired flatfoot deformity, and all practitioners should be able to quickly diagnose it and be familiar with its treatment. Although an entire textbook could be dedicated to this topic, this article briefly summarizes classic presentation, diagnostic principles, and nonsurgical treatment option.

Presentation

The most common form of PTT dysfunction is degeneration of the tendon in its watershed region distal to the medial malleolus, although the cause behind this remains unknown.[16–18] Although acute ruptures of the PTT are known to occur, most often in the setting of an ankle fracture, these remain rare.[19–21] PTT dysfunction is most common in women older than the age of 50. It can be associated with several underlying disorders, including diabetes, obesity, previous surgery or trauma in the area, steroid injections, and inflammatory conditions.[10,17–20]

The disease process is progressive, starting with PTT tenosynovitis, in which patients may complain of pain posterior to and distal to the medial malleolus. As the disease progresses, the patient may complain that they are becoming flat-footed and have difficulty standing on their toes on the effected side. As the disease progresses to its characteristic collapse of the medial arch with hindfoot valgus and forefoot abduction and varus, the patient may develop painful symptoms secondary to subtalar and ultimately tibiotalar arthritis.[18,22]

DIAGNOSIS
Physical Examination/Staging

Stage 1 presents with medial pain along the PTT. Physical examination may demonstrate swelling and warmth along the tendon. The patient may be tender just posterior and distal to the medial malleolus. At this stage, there is no deformity, and motor strength is retained, as is flexibility. The patient should still be able to perform a single limb heel raise.[16,17,22–24]

Stage 2 is characterized by the progression to hindfoot valgus with possible forefoot abduction. The foot remains flexible, and the examiner can correct both the hindfoot valgus and the forefoot abduction. The patient may have difficulty or be unable to perform a single-limb heel raise. Upon standing, the examiner can observe the hindfoot valgus as well as the forefoot abduction and varus ("too many toes" sign). Looking medially, the examiner will notice a collapse of the arch.[16,22]

Stage 3 is the progression to a rigid deformity with fixed forefoot abduction. Attempts at reducing the hindfoot will uncover forefoot supination. The subtalar joint is frequently arthritic, and the patient is unable to perform a single-limb heal raise. Often there is no medial-sided pain over the PTT, and pain is limited to the arthritic subtalar joint and lateral side secondary to subfibular impingement. The examiner may observe wrinkles in the lateral foot secondary to redundant skin. The gastroc-soleus should be evaluated, as it is tight at this stage of the disease.[17,18,22,25]

Stage 4 is the progression of the disease to the ankle joint. Eccentric valgus loading of the tibiotalar joint leads to an incongruent valgus deformity of the talus in the mortise. Lateral pain is present secondary both ankle arthritis and subfibular impingement.[26,27]

Imaging

Radiographs are integral in the evaluation of PTT dysfunction. Plain films may demonstrate a loss of the normal Meary (talar-first metatarsal) angle, loss of calcaneal pitch, peritalar subluxation, and talar-navicular uncoverage. At later stages, radiographs may demonstrate talar tilt and subtalar/tibiotalar arthritis.[22,28–30]

Ultrasound has been used to evaluate PTT dysfunction. Ultrasound can demonstrate fluid about the tendon in tenosynovitis. It can also show longitudinal tears of the PTT or absence of the tendon in its groove in the case of ruptures.[31]

MRI can evaluate all stages of PTT dysfunction. It will demonstrate fluid within the tendon sheath and tendon hypertrophy in stage 1. In stage 2 and 3, MRI will reveal tendon elongation and split tears and ultimately complete rupture. MRI has also been used to evaluate the spring ligament.[14,32–34]

NONSURGICAL TREATMENT OPTIONS

Although surgical intervention has become commonplace for all stages of PTT dysfunction, nonsurgical treatment is also possible at all stages. In addition, a trial of nonsurgical treatment should also be implemented before surgery. Treatment of stage 1 and 2 PTT dysfunction is aimed at correcting the deformity to stop progression of the disease, whereas treatment of stage 3 and 4 disease is aimed at symptom relief and holding the deformity in situ to slow progression.[35–38]

Early PTT dysfunction/tenosynovitis may be initially treated with a period of immobilization with nonsteroidal anti-inflammatory medications (NSAIDs), depending on the patient's tolerance of these medications. The level of immobilization ranges from casting to a walking boot, to rigid stirrup or lace up brace depending on practitioner preference. Once the patient's pain subsides, they should be fit with custom-molded in-shoe orthosis.[36,38] If unable to tolerate an in-shoe orthosis, they should be fit with a molded AFO. They should also start physical therapy for strengthening of the PTT as well as stretching of the gastroc-soleus complex.

In later stages where the hindfoot has become rigid, orthotics aimed at correcting the deformity is no longer useful. For these stages, molded AFOs or Arizona braces are required to hold the deformity in situ.[35,36,38,39] The aim is to provide symptomatic relief and allow the patient an acceptable degree of function. Bracing may also slow the progression of the disease. Obviously, failure of these modalities to provide symptomatic relief may require surgical intervention.

ACHILLES TENDON

Achilles tendonitis and ruptures are commonly encountered and affect athletes and nonathletes alike. Although literature on the subject has been controversial, most conditions may be treated nonsurgically. Recent studies have suggested an increase in the incidence of Achilles ruptures, requiring all practitioners to be comfortable treating these injuries.[40–43]

PRESENTATION

Achilles tendon abnormalities affect all genders and ages; however, acute ruptures are mostly in men in their fourth and fifth decades of life involved in athletic activity.[41–44] Although repetitive use is common to all abnormalities, many associated conditions have been implicated in Achilles tendinopathy, including obesity, hypertension, systemic disease (lupus, anklyosing spondylitis), steroid use, hormone replacement, or fluoroquinolone use.[44–46]

Pain is the primary complaint in all Achilles tendon disorders. Pain is usually associated with activity, although it may also be increased in the morning.[47] In acute tendonitis, the patient may report a recent increase in activity level or change in activity type. Chronic tendinopathy must be divided into insertional and noninsertional type and is characterized by the location of the patient's pain. Each involves a degenerative condition, but midsubstance pain typically occurs 2 to 6 cm above the Achilles insertion, whereas the insertional type occurs directly at the insertion.[46–48] Insertional Achilles tendonitis patients may complain of more pain with certain shoe wear.

Acute ruptures usually present with a history of recent sports injury. Commonly, the patient will describe an acute "pop" during activity and a feeling as though they were struck or shot from behind. This feeling is followed by immediate pain and inability to bear weight and difficulty with plantarflexion.[44,49–51]

DIAGNOSIS
Physical Examination

The physical examination should reliably allow the examiner to diagnose the type of Achilles abnormality in each patient. Inspection may reveal atrophy of the gastroc-soleus complex compared with the contralateral leg or may demonstrate swelling, erythema, or prominence over the symptomatic area. In acute ruptures, significant ecchymosis may be apparent on examination. Palpation will allow the examiner to hone in on the symptomatic region as well as assess the contour of the tendon itself. Any defects or nodules should be noted. Midsubstance tendinopathy and ruptures typically report pain with palpation 2 to 6 cm proximal to the insertion, whereas insertional tendinopathy will elicit pain directly over the insertion. Acute tendonitis may have a more generalized area of tenderness along the tendon. To ensure the tendon is intact, a Thompson test should be performed. In addition, an examination of resting tension will reveal that the affected extremity will rest in a position of decreased plantarflexion compared with the well leg. If the tendon is intact, the examiner may proceed with motor strength testing or ask the patient to perform single-leg heel raises.

Imaging

Although many of these disorders may be diagnosed by physical examination alone, radiographic evaluation is often helpful, especially in incomplete tears or tendinopathy. A lateral radiograph may often demonstrate a Haglund deformity in the setting of insertional tendinopathy.[48] Ultrasound and MRI have both been used to assess ruptures of the Achilles as well as tendinopathies. Ultrasound is cost-effective and has been used to diagnose many conditions, but it remains user-dependent and is unreliable in differentiating partial tears from other focal lesions.[52–54] Although expensive and often unnecessary, MRI allows higher-resolution assessment and increases the ability to differentiate among tendinopathies and to evaluate partial ruptures, tumors, and healing of the Achilles tendon.[33,55,56]

NONSURGICAL TREATMENT

All Achilles disorders may be treated nonsurgically, including acute ruptures. The initial management of both insertional and noninsertional tendinopathy is the same. Activity modification is the cornerstone of treatment, and inciting activities should be avoided.[46–48] Activity modification may be preceded by a short period of immobilization in cast or boot with or without a heel lift. NSAIDs may be helpful for symptom relief.[57] Once symptoms have subsided, the patient should begin physical therapy with eccentric strengthening and stretching.[47] Physical therapy may be supplemented with other modalities, including ultrasound, extracorporeal shock wave therapy, iontophoresis, and phonophoresis.[53,58] Night splinting may be added to eccentric exercises to help with residual symptoms, but efficacy is controversial.[59] As with other tendon disorders, steroid injections should be avoided because of its association with rupture.

Achilles ruptures may also be treated nonsurgically, and many studies have shown similar results to surgical intervention. Although nonsurgical treatment is cost-effective and eliminates the concern of surgical complications, it does have significantly higher rates of rerupture and may not be appropriate for the younger and more active patient.[41,42,50,51] Although technique and length of immobilization are debated, the treatment typically consists of 6 to 8 weeks of immobilization of the affected leg in resting gravity equinus to approximate the ruptured ends of the tendon and allow them to heal. Newer studies suggest that short periods of immobilization with early functional rehabilitation protocols may be beneficial and lead to rerupture rates closer to that of surgically treated ruptures.[51,60]

PERONEAL TENDONS

Although complete rupture of the peroneal tendons is rare, the tendons are prone to tendonitis, tearing, and subluxation/dislocation. They can be a source of lateral ankle pain and may occur in the setting of instability. The physician must be able to differentiate from other sources of lateral ankle pain.

PRESENTATION

Posterolateral ankle pain is the most common complaint of those patients presenting with peroneal disorders. Those presenting with tendinitis may complain of insidious onset of swelling and pain note that their symptoms are activity related. They may report a recent change in activity level or type.[61] However, peroneal tendon disorders are frequently found in the setting of ankle instability, so the patient may report a history of inversion injury or chronic sprains.[62] They may recall an acute "pop" as with Achilles tendon injuries followed by pain and swelling. In more chronic cases, the incident may not be well defined, and a careful history to elicit symptoms of instability versus pain must be taken. Patients with subluxation may complain of painful clicking.[61,63] Individuals with a varus hindfoot or shallow fibular groove are also more prone to peroneal disorders. Although a rare presentation, one must also recognize that a tear of the superior peroneal retinaculum may go unnoticed in the setting of a calcaneus fracture. These are difficult to diagnose secondary to pain and inability to test for peroneal instability. Unfortunately, unless recognized during surgery, this is more often than not a delayed presentation of peroneal tendon abnormality.

DIAGNOSIS
Physical Examination

Inspection may reveal swelling over the peroneal tendons. In the setting of an acute injury, ecchymosis may be present. Hindfoot and forefoot alignment should be noted. Palpation will reveal tenderness over the course of the tendons, and it may be possible to palpate thickening of the tendons. Stability of the ankle should be thoroughly assessed. If the peroneal tendons are unstable, it may be possible to appreciate the subluxation with dorsiflexion/plantarflexion along with resisted eversion.[61] If only one peroneal tendon is affected, motor testing may appear normal, because the remaining peroneal is able to compensate during resisted eversion.

Imaging

Radiographs should be obtained for those presenting with lateral ankle pain. Talar osteochondral lesions or fibular avulsion fractures may be noted in the presence of instability and peroneal abnormality.[64] An os peroneum may also be present and contributieto the symptoms. However, often the radiographs will be negative in the setting of isolated peroneal disorders. As with the other tendons of the ankle, ultrasonography is useful in the evaluation of peroneal tendon abnormality and may demonstrate edema, tendon thickening, and disruption.[65,66] Ultrasound may be most helpful in the dynamic evaluation of peroneal subluxation.[67] MRI provides the most detail regarding tendon abnormality and is very useful in evaluating longitudinal split tears.[34,61,66] In addition, an MRI can simultaneously evaluate the integrity of the retinaculum, depth of the fibular groove, presence of osteochondral lesions of the talus, and other coexistent abnormalities.

NONSURGICAL TREATMENT

Conservative treatment of peroneal tendon abnormality is similar to that of the other tendons of the ankle and can be very effective. A short period (3–4 weeks) of immobilization in a cast or boot can be useful in settling down symptoms.[61,63,68] NSAIDs may be used to help with inflammation and pain. Following symptomatic improvement, physical therapy may be prescribed to help with strengthening and range of motion. Activity modification should focus on reducing or eliminating activities that previously produced painful symptoms.[61,64,69] If varus alignment of the hindfoot is present, a lateral heel wedge may be trialed. Local injections of steroids have been used effectively, but the use of steroids should be used carefully, and the ankle should be protected to prevent rupture.[10,69] Recent studies have shown improvement in symptoms following local platelet-rich plasma injections of the tendons of the ankle.[70]

REFERENCES

1. Anagnostakos K, Bachelier F, Fürst OA, et al. Rupture of the anterior tibial tendon: three clinical cases, anatomical study, and literature review. Foot Ankle Int 2006; 27:330–9.
2. Anon. Injuries of the extensor tendons in the distal part of the I...: JBJS. LWW. Available at: http://journals.lww.com/jbjsjournal/Fulltext/1955/37060/INJURIES_OF_THE_EXTENSOR_TENDONS_IN_THE_DISTAL.7.aspx. Accessed March 4, 2017.
3. Beischer AD, Beamond BM, Jowett AJL, et al. Distal tendinosis of the tibialis anterior tendon. Foot Ankle Int 2009;30:1053–9.
4. Grundy JRB, O'Sullivan RM, Beischer AD. Operative management of distal tibialis anterior tendinopathy. Foot Ankle Int 2010;31:212–9.
5. Gwynne-Jones D, Garneti N, Wyatt M. Closed tibialis anterior tendon rupture: a case series. Foot Ankle Int 2009;30:758–62.
6. Markarian GG, Kelikian AS, Brage M, et al. Anterior tibialis tendon ruptures: an outcome analysis of operative versus nonoperative treatment. Foot Ankle Int 1998;19:792–802.
7. Mechrefe AP, Walsh EF, DiGiovanni CW. Anterior tibial tendon avulsion with distal tibial fracture entrapment: case report. Foot Ankle Int 2006;27:645–7.
8. Ouzounian TJ, Anderson R. Anterior tibial tendon rupture. Foot Ankle Int 1995;16: 406–10.
9. Patten A, Pun W-K. Spontaneous rupture of the tibialis anterior tendon: a case report and literature review. Foot Ankle Int 2000;21:697–700.
10. Ford LT, DeBender J. Tendon rupture after local steroid injection. South Med J 1979;72:827–30.
11. Jerome JTJ, Varghese M, Sankaran B, et al. Tibialis anterior tendon rupture in gout–case report and literature review. Foot Ankle Surg 2008;14:166–9.
12. Mirza MA, Korber KE. Isolated rupture of the tibialis anterior tendon associated with a fracture of the tibial shaft: a case report. Orthopedics 1984;7:1329–32.
13. Peetrons P. Lesions of the anterior tibial tendon using ultrasonography: report of 2 cases. JBR-BTR 1999;82:157–8 [in French].
14. Kier R, Dietz MJ, McCarthy SM, et al. MR imaging of the normal ligaments and tendons of the ankle. J Comput Assist Tomogr 1991;15:477–82.
15. Mengiardi B, Pfirrmann CWA, Vienne P, et al. Anterior tibial tendon abnormalities: MR imaging findings. Radiology 2005;235:977–84.
16. Beals TC, Pomeroy GC, Manoli A. Posterior tibial tendon insufficiency: diagnosis and treatment. J Am Acad Orthop Surg 1999;7:112–8.
17. Geideman WM, Johnson JE. Posterior tibial tendon dysfunction. J Orthop Sports Phys Ther 2000;30:68–77.
18. Giza E, Cush G, Schon LC. The flexible flatfoot in the adult. Foot Ankle Clin 2007; 12:251–71, vi.
19. Bernstein DT, Harris JD, Cosculluela PE, et al. Acute tibialis posterior tendon rupture with pronation-type ankle fractures. Orthopedics 2016;39:e970–5.

20. DeMill SL, Bussewitz BW, Philbin TM. Injury to the posterior tibial tendon after open reduction internal fixation of the medial malleolus. Foot Ankle Spec 2015; 8:360–3.

21. Martinelli N, Bonifacini C, Bianchi A, et al. Acute rupture of the tibialis posterior tendon without fracture: a case report. J Am Podiatr Med Assoc 2014;104: 298–301.

22. Abousayed MM, Tartaglione JP, Rosenbaum AJ, et al. Classifications in brief: Johnson and Strom classification of adult-acquired flatfoot deformity. Clin Orthop 2016;474:588–93.

23. Bare AA, Haddad SL. Tenosynovitis of the posterior tibial tendon. Foot Ankle Clin 2001;6:37–66.

24. Funk DA, Cass JR, Johnson KA. Acquired adult flat foot secondary to posterior tibial-tendon abnormality. J Bone Joint Surg Am 1986;68:95–102.

25. Raikin SM, Winters BS, Daniel JN. The RAM classification: a novel, systematic approach to the adult-acquired flatfoot. Foot Ankle Clin 2012;17:169–81.

26. Bluman EM, Myerson MS. Stage IV posterior tibial tendon rupture. Foot Ankle Clin 2007;12:341–62, viii.

27. Bohay DR, Anderson JG. Stage IV posterior tibial tendon insufficiency: the tilted ankle. Foot Ankle Clin 2003;8:619–36.

28. Meehan RE, Brage M. Adult acquired flat foot deformity: clinical and radiographic examination. Foot Ankle Clin 2003;8:431–52.

29. Sensiba PR, Coffey MJ, Williams NE, et al. Inter- and intraobserver reliability in the radiographic evaluation of adult flatfoot deformity. Foot Ankle Int 2010;31:141–5.

30. Younger AS, Sawatzky B, Dryden P. Radiographic assessment of adult flatfoot. Foot Ankle Int 2005;26:820–5.

31. Premkumar A, Perry MB, Dwyer AJ, et al. Sonography and MR imaging of posterior tibial tendinopathy. AJR Am J Roentgenol 2002;178:223–32.

32. Feighan J, Towers J, Conti S. The use of magnetic resonance imaging in posterior tibial tendon dysfunction. Clin Orthop 1999;(365):23–38.

33. Peduto AJ, Read JW. Imaging of ankle tendinopathy and tears. Top Magn Reson Imaging 2010;21:25–36.

34. Schweitzer ME, Karasick D. MRI of the ankle and hindfoot. Semin Ultrasound CT MR 1994;15:410–22.

35. Augustin JF, Lin SS, Berberian WS, et al. Nonoperative treatment of adult acquired flat foot with the Arizona brace. Foot Ankle Clin 2003;8:491–502.

36. Chao W, Wapner KL, Lee TH, et al. Nonoperative management of posterior tibial tendon dysfunction. Foot Ankle Int 1996;17:736–41.

37. Nielsen MD, Dodson EE, Shadrick DL, et al. Nonoperative care for the treatment of adult-acquired flatfoot deformity. J Foot Ankle Surg 2011;50:311–4.

38. Wapner KL, Chao W. Nonoperative treatment of posterior tibial tendon dysfunction. Clin Orthop 1999;(365):39–45.

39. Noll KH. The use of orthotic devices in adult acquired flatfoot deformity. Foot Ankle Clin 2001;6:25–36.

40. Bradley JP, Tibone JE. Percutaneous and open surgical repairs of Achilles tendon ruptures. A comparative study. Am J Sports Med 1990;18:188–95.

41. Ganestam A, Kallemose T, Troelsen A, et al. Increasing incidence of acute Achilles tendon rupture and a noticeable decline in surgical treatment from 1994 to 2013. A nationwide registry study of 33,160 patients. Knee Surg Sports Traumatol Arthrosc 2016;24(12):3730–7.

42. Gwynne-Jones DP, Sims M, Handcock D. Epidemiology and outcomes of acute Achilles tendon rupture with operative or nonoperative treatment using an identical functional bracing protocol. Foot Ankle Int 2011;32:337–43.

43. Huttunen TT, Kannus P, Rolf C, et al. Acute achilles tendon ruptures: incidence of injury and surgery in Sweden between 2001 and 2012. Am J Sports Med 2014; 42:2419–23.

44. Claessen FMAP, de Vos R-J, Reijman M, et al. Predictors of primary Achilles tendon ruptures. Sports Med 2014;44:1241–59.

45. Järvinen TAH, Kannus P, Maffulli N, et al. Achilles tendon disorders: etiology and epidemiology. Foot Ankle Clin 2005;10:255–66.

46. Longo UG, Ronga M, Maffulli N. Achilles tendinopathy. Sports Med Arthrosc 2009;17:112–26.

47. Weinfeld SB. Achilles tendon disorders. Med Clin North Am 2014;98:331–8.

48. Irwin TA. Current concepts review: insertional achilles tendinopathy. Foot Ankle Int 2010;31:933–9.

49. Longo UG, Petrillo S, Maffulli N, et al. Acute achilles tendon rupture in athletes. Foot Ankle Clin 2013;18:319–38.

50. Ronninger CH, Kuhn K, Follaro T, et al. Operative and nonoperative management of Achilles tendon ruptures in active duty military population. Foot Ankle Int 2016; 37:269–73.

51. Willits K, Amendola A, Bryant D, et al. Operative versus nonoperative treatment of acute Achilles tendon ruptures: a multicenter randomized trial using accelerated functional rehabilitation. J Bone Joint Surg Am 2010;92:2767–75.

52. Carroll M, Dalbeth N, Boocock M, et al. The assessment of lesions of the Achilles tendon by ultrasound imaging in inflammatory arthritis: a systematic review and meta-analysis. Semin Arthritis Rheum 2015;45:103–14.

53. Daftary A, Adler RS. Sonographic evaluation and ultrasound-guided therapy of the Achilles tendon. Ultrasound Q 2009;25:103–10.

54. Paavola M, Paakkala T, Kannus P, et al. Ultrasonography in the differential diagnosis of Achilles tendon injuries and related disorders. A comparison between pre-operative ultrasonography and surgical findings. Acta Radiol 1998;39:612–9.

55. Panageas E, Greenberg S, Franklin PD, et al. Magnetic resonance imaging of pathologic conditions of the Achilles tendon. Orthop Rev 1990;19:975–80.

56. Pierre-Jerome C, Moncayo V, Terk MR. MRI of the Achilles tendon: a comprehensive review of the anatomy, biomechanics, and imaging of overuse tendinopathies. Acta Radiol 2010;51:438–54.

57. McLauchlan GJ, Handoll HH. Interventions for treating acute and chronic Achilles tendinitis. Cochrane Database Syst Rev 2001;(2):CD000232.

58. Al-Abbad H, Simon JV. The effectiveness of extracorporeal shock wave therapy on chronic achilles tendinopathy: a systematic review. Foot Ankle Int 2013;34: 33–41.

59. De Vos RJ, Weir A, Visser RJA, et al. The additional value of a night splint to eccentric exercises in chronic midportion Achilles tendinopathy: a randomised controlled trial. Br J Sports Med 2007;41:e5.

60. Barfod KW, Bencke J, Lauridsen HB, et al. Nonoperative dynamic treatment of acute achilles tendon rupture: the influence of early weight-bearing on clinical outcome: a blinded, randomized controlled trial. J Bone Joint Surg Am 2014; 96:1497–503.

61. Roster B, Michelier P, Giza E. Peroneal tendon disorders. Clin Sports Med 2015; 34:625–41.

62. DiGiovanni BF, Fraga CJ, Cohen BE, et al. Associated injuries found in chronic lateral ankle instability. Foot Ankle Int 2000;21:809–15.
63. Dombek MF, Lamm BM, Saltrick K, et al. Peroneal tendon tears: a retrospective review. J Foot Ankle Surg 2003;42:250–8.
64. Baumhauer JF, Nawoczenski DA, DiGiovanni BF, et al. Ankle pain and peroneal tendon pathology. Clin Sports Med 2004;23:21–34.
65. Bianchi S, Delmi M, Molini L. Ultrasound of peroneal tendons. Semin Musculoskelet Radiol 2010;14:292–306.
66. Lee SJ, Jacobson JA, Kim S-M, et al. Ultrasound and MRI of the peroneal tendons and associated pathology. Skeletal Radiol 2013;42:1191–200.
67. Pesquer L, Guillo S, Poussange N, et al. Dynamic ultrasound of peroneal tendon instability. Br J Radiol 2016;89:20150958.
68. McLennan JG. Treatment of acute and chronic luxations of the peroneal tendons. Am J Sports Med 1980;8:432–6.
69. Philbin TM, Landis GS, Smith B. Peroneal tendon injuries. J Am Acad Orthop Surg 2009;17:306–17.
70. Dallaudière B, Pesquer L, Meyer P, et al. Intratendinous injection of platelet-rich plasma under US guidance to treat tendinopathy: a long-term pilot study. J Vasc Interv Radiol 2014;25:717–23.

The Acute Injury of the Achilles

Surgical Options (Open Treatment, and, Minimally Invasive Surgery)

Oliver Schipper, MD[a,b,]*, Bruce Cohen, MD[a]

KEYWORDS

• Achilles rupture • Achilles repair • Achilles tendinitis

KEY POINTS

- Achilles tendon rupture is a common lower extremity injury seen in the active population.
- Although reruptures rates have improved with nonoperative functional management, the authors still prefer surgical treatment.
- Percutaneous, minimally invasive procedures may allow optimal Achilles tendon rupture apposition and tensioning, with a reduced risk of soft tissue complications associated with the traditional open repair.

INTRODUCTION

Acute Achilles injuries (<6 weeks) are common in the lower extremity and typically occur in the midsubstance tendinous portion of the gastrocnemius-soleus tendon complex but may also occur proximally at the myotendinous junction or at the insertion as an Achilles sleeve avulsion. Incidence is highest in men aged 30 to 39 years.[1–3] The predominant mechanism is indirect, secondary to forced ankle dorsiflexion against a contracted gastrocnemius-soleus complex. Treatment options vary based on the level of rupture.

Historically, nonoperative, non–weight-bearing immobilization for acute Achilles ruptures had clinically inferior outcomes compared with surgical management, specifically with regard to rerupture rate.[4] With the advent of functional nonoperative rehabilitation with early weight bearing, management of acute midsubstance Achilles ruptures is no longer as clear-cut. A randomized multicenter trial comparing open

[a] OrthoCarolina Foot and Ankle Institute, 2001 Vail Avenue, Suite 200B, Charlotte, NC 28207, USA; [b] Anderson Orthopaedic Clinic, 2445 Army Navy Drive, Arlington, Virginia 22206, USA
* Corresponding author. Anderson Orthopaedic Clinic, 2445 Army Navy Drive, Arlington, Virginia 22206.
E-mail address: o.schipper@gmail.com

Foot Ankle Clin N Am 22 (2017) 689–714
http://dx.doi.org/10.1016/j.fcl.2017.07.003
1083-7515/17/© 2017 Elsevier Inc. All rights reserved.

foot.theclinics.com

surgical Achilles tendon repair with nonoperative accelerated functional rehabilitation showed no significant difference with a minimum 2-year follow-up with respect to rerupture rate, clinical outcomes, strength, and calf circumference. The study was underpowered to determine a true difference in rerupture rate.[5] Also, it showed significantly higher plantar flexion strength at the 240°/s test velocity and soft tissue complications in the operative group. Thus, nonoperative functional rehabilitation with early weight bearing is an acceptable form of management for acute Achilles ruptures, although further randomized controlled trials are necessary to further delineate the differences between operative and nonoperative management. Regardless of treatment, early functional rehabilitation and weight bearing seem to play an important role in successful outcomes after acute Achilles tendon rupture (**Box 1**). If a patient presents greater than 6 weeks after rupture, nonoperative management is recommended unless there is evidence of significant retraction of the proximal stump on imaging.

In an effort to reduce soft tissue complications, the trend for operative management has been toward minimally invasive techniques and away from the traditional open technique. Ma and Griffith[6] initially described a percutaneous technique in 1977 using small stab incisions along the border of the Achilles tendon, which was subsequently modified to increase the strength of the repair and avoid sural nerve entrapment.[6,7] A prospective randomized controlled trial with minimum 6-month follow-up comparing the traditional open technique with the modified Ma and Griffith[6] percutaneous technique showed a significant reduction in wound complications and only a 3% incidence of persistent sural nerve paresthesia in the percutaneous group.[8] Kakiuchi[9] subsequently described a combined miniopen, percutaneous technique in order to better evaluate the tendon stump apposition and minimize wound complications. This technique was used as the foundation for the modern Achillon System and Percutaneous Achilles Repair System (PARS) techniques using an instrumented jig to place the sutures within the tendon sheath. Initial outcomes using the Achillon jig for acute Achilles tendon repair were encouraging, with no wound problems or sural nerve disturbances reported in 87 consecutive patients at a mean follow-up of 26 months.[10] There were 3 reruptures secondary to noncompliance and a fall. In a more recent study of early surgical outcomes after acute Achilles rupture comparing the open technique with the PARS, there were no significant differences in the rate of rerupture, sural nerve paresthesia, wound dehiscence, or reoperation.[11] No power analysis was performed and the study used a minimum 3-month follow-up, so little information can be drawn with regard to rerupture rates. Another comparison of open and percutaneous repairs showed significantly fewer major complications in the percutaneous group, particularly wound necrosis, and a lower total number of complications.[12] There was no significant difference in sural nerve disturbances.

Little evidence exists to guide management of proximal myotendinous Achilles ruptures. A retrospective case series of 30 myotendinous Achilles ruptures in patients with a mean age of 40.5 years managed nonoperatively showed significant improvement in both mean Foot and Ankle Ability Measure–Sports and visual analog scale scores. There were no Achilles reruptures at a mean of 40.5 months.[13]

Similarly, outcomes after management of Achilles insertional tendon sleeve avulsions are poorly described. Preexisting Achilles tendinosis is often present as well as an associated Haglund deformity. A retrospective case series of 11 patients managed operatively with suture anchor repair showed excellent results with only 1 complication (delayed wound healing).[14]

Box 1
Accelerated rehabilitation program for nonoperative treatment of Achilles tendon ruptures

- 0 to 2 weeks
  - Plaster cast with ankle plantar flexed approximately 20° non–weight bearing with crutches
- 2 to 4 weeks
  - Walking boot with 2-cm to 4-cm heel lift
  - Protected weight bearing with crutches:
    - Week 2 to 3: 25%
    - Week 3 to 4: 50%
    - Week 4 to 5: 75%
    - Week 5 to 6: 100%
  - Active plantar and dorsiflexion range-of-motion exercises to neutral, inversion/eversion below neutral
  - Modalities to control swelling (ultrasonography, acupuncture, light/laser therapy)
  - Electromuscular stimulation to calf musculature with seated heel raises when tolerated
  - Patients being seen 2 to 3 times per week depending on availability and degree of pain and swelling in the foot and ankle
  - Non–weight-bearing fitness/cardiovascular work; for example, biking with 1 leg (with walker boot on), deep-water running
  - Emphasize need for patient to use pain as a guideline if in pain, back off activities and weight bearing
- 4 to 6 weeks
  - Advance activities and weight bearing
  - Ensure that ankle does not go past neutral while doing exercises
  - Emphasize patient doing non–weight-bearing cardiovascular activities as tolerated with boot walker on
- 6 to 8 weeks
  - Continue physical therapy 2 times a week
  - Continue with modalities for swelling as needed
  - Continue with EMS on calf with strengthening exercises; do not go past neutral ankle position
  - Remove heel lift (if had two 2-cm lifts, take 1 out at a time over 2–3 days)
  - Weight bearing as tolerated, usually 100% weight bearing in boot walker at this time
  - Active assisted dorsiflexion stretching, slowly initially with a belt in sitting position
  - Graduated resistance exercises (open and closed kinetic chain as well as functional activities); start with Theraband exercises
  - With weighted resistance exercises, do not go past neutral ankle position
  - Gait retraining now that patient is 100% weight bearing
  - Fitness/cardiovascular work to include weight bearing as tolerated; for example, biking
  - Hydrotherapy
- 8 to 12 weeks
  - Ensure patient understands that tendon is still vulnerable and patients need to be diligent with activities of daily living and exercises; any sudden loading of the Achilles (eg, trip, step up stairs) may result in a rerupture
  - Wean off boot (usually over 2–5 days but varies between patients)
  - Return to crutches/cane as necessary and gradually wean off
  - Continue to progress range-of-motion, strength, proprioception exercises
  - Add exercises such as stationary bicycle, elliptical bicycle, walking on treadmill as patient tolerates
  - Add wobble board activities; progress from seated to supported standing to standing as tolerated
  - Add calf stretches in standing position (gently)
    - Do not allow ankle to go past neutral position
  - Add double heel raises and progress to single heel raises when tolerated
    - Do not allow ankle to go past neutral position
  - Continue physical therapy 1 to 2 times a week depending on how independent patient is at doing exercises and whether patient has access to exercise equipment

- 12 to 16 weeks
  - Physical therapy 1 to 2 times a week
  - Retrain strength, power, endurance through eccentric strengthening exercises and closed kinetic chain exercises
- 16 weeks plus
  - Increase dynamic weight-bearing exercise, including sport-specific retraining; that is, jogging, weight training
- 4 to 6 months
  - Return to normal sporting activities that do not involve contact or sprinting, cutting, jumping, and so forth if patient has regained 80% strength
- 6 to 9 months
  - Return to sports that involve running/jumping as directed by medical team and tolerated if patient has regained 100% strength

Data from Willits K, Amendola A, Bryant D, et al. Operative versus nonoperative treatment of acute Achilles tendon ruptures: a multicenter randomized trial using accelerated functional rehabilitation. J Bone Joint Surg Am 2010;92(17):2767–75.

PATIENT EVALUATION OVERVIEW
Patient History

- May report sudden pain and swelling in posterior ankle with forced dorsiflexion of contracted plantar flexed foot
- May experience pop in posterior ankle
- Ask about any paresthesias in the foot present before or after the injury
- May have inability to bear weight or weakness with push-off during gait
- Question about history of preceding Achilles tendinitis/tendinosis, corticosteroid injection, or fluoroquinolone use

Patient Physical Examination (American Academy of Orthopaedic Surgery Clinical Practice Guidelines)

- Examine for posterior ankle edema and ecchymosis[15]
- Perform a thorough neurovascular examination, including examination for palpable pulses and neurologic examination with particular attention paid to the sural nerve
- With the patient prone, palpate from proximal myotendinous region through distal Achilles tendon insertion for tenderness and appreciable gap in tendon
- Examine for decreased ankle plantar flexion strength and increased passive ankle dorsiflexion with gentle manipulation
- Perform Thompson test:
  - With the patient prone, squeeze the proximal calf
  - Positive test if no plantar flexion of the ankle
  - If equivocal, can compare with the other side for asymmetry
- Perform knee flexion test
  - With the patient prone, flex both knees to 90° and examine the resting position of both ankles
  - Positive test if asymmetry of resting position of both ankles with the less plantar flexed ankle being positive for Achilles rupture

Imaging

- Lateral ankle radiograph is not required, but may see soft tissue defect in Achilles tendon, or small piece of bone within Achilles tendon concerning for Achilles tendon insertional sleeve avulsion (**Fig. 1**).

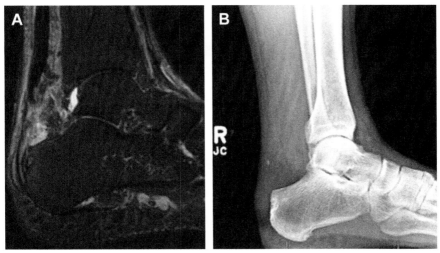

Fig. 1. MRI without contrast (*A*) and radiograph (*B*) showing evidence of insertional Achilles rupture. On radiograph, a small bony fragment can be seen proximal to the tendon insertion, signifying rupture from donor Achilles insertion site.

- MRI is not required but may be obtained if equivocal physical examination or if unable to determine level of rupture for surgical planning.
- Ultrasonography is low cost and may be performed in the office. In the sagittal plane, a hypoechoic gap in Achilles tendon may be appreciated if rupture is present. The tendon should otherwise be uniform in echogenicity.
  - A real-time Achilles Ultrasonography Thompson test can be performed in which the examiner performs a Thompson test under ultrasonography (86.4% sensitivity, 91.7% specificity for Achilles tendon rupture).[16]

SURGICAL TREATMENT OPTIONS FOR MIDSUBSTANCE ACHILLES TENDON RUPTURE
Traditional Open Technique

- Indications:
  - Primary repair of an acute (<6 weeks) Achilles midsubstance tendon rupture
  - Repair of a failed miniopen or percutaneous Achilles repair
  - Adequate soft tissue envelope amenable to a traditional open Achilles incision
- Equipment:
  - No. 2 nonabsorbable braided suture
- Positioning:
  - Performed with patient prone under general anesthesia with optional popliteal pain catheter for postoperative analgesia
  - Thigh tourniquet placed
  - (Optional) can drape out both legs to compare resting tension of contralateral Achilles tendon
- Surgical approach:
  - A 5-cm to 8-cm longitudinal posteromedial incision is made centered on the rupture site (**Fig. 2**)
    - The richest vascular zones are located medially and laterally to the Achilles tendon compared with the midline posterior vascular zone[17]

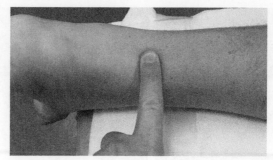

Fig. 2. A 5-cm to 8-cm longitudinal posteromedial incision is made, centered on the rupture site.

- ○ Paratenon is incised and elevated (**Fig. 3**)
  - ■ Used for closure after Achilles tendon repair
- ○ Achilles rupture is identified (**Fig. 4**)
- ○ No. 2 suture is placed in a Krackow suture configuration into each end of the ruptured tendon (**Fig. 5**)
  - ■ Modified Bunnell, Kessler, and triple-bundle suture techniques have also been described
  - ■ Triple-bundle technique is biomechanically stronger (2.8 times) than the Krackow technique but carries a higher suture burden[18]
  - ■ Gift-box modification of the Krackow suture has also been described and has shown a 2-fold increase in pull-out strength compared with the traditional Krackow suture technique[19]
- ○ Tendon ends are reapproximated and secured using a 2-strand construct (**Fig. 6**)
- ○ Repair site is reinforced running epitendinous suture (3-0 nonbraided suture)
- ○ Paratenon is then closed with a 2-0 running Vicryl suture
- ○ Subcutaneous tissue is closed with 3-0 Monocryl
- ○ Skin is closed with 3-0 nylon sutures

Minimally Invasive Technique Using the Achillon

- • Indications:
  - ○ Primary repair of an acute (<3–4 weeks) Achilles tendon rupture occurring between 2 cm and 8 cm proximal to the calcaneal tuberosity
    - ■ Primary repair of tears that are 3 to 6 weeks old may also be performed but require release of scar tissue adhesions between the tendon and paratenon in order to adequately mobilize the tendon ends for apposition

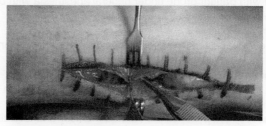

Fig. 3. Paratenon is incised and elevated.

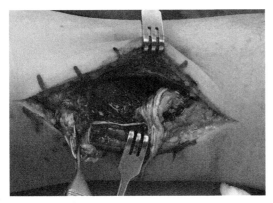

Fig. 4. Achilles rupture is identified.

- ○ Contraindications include chronic ruptures greater than 6 weeks old, prior Achilles surgery, and open ruptures secondary to laceration
- Equipment:
  - ○ Achillon System (Integra)
- Positioning:
  - ○ Performed with patient prone under general anesthesia with optional popliteal pain catheter for postoperative analgesia
  - ○ Thigh tourniquet placed
  - ○ (Optional) can drape out both legs to compare resting tension of contralateral Achilles tendon
- Surgical approach:
  - ○ Medial longitudinal incision is made 1.5 to 2 cm in length extending proximally from the palpable tendon defect
  - ○ A 2-cm incision is made in the paratenon
  - ○ Finger dissection is used to free the proximal and distal tendon stumps from the paratenon
  - ○ The proximal stump is grasped with an Allis clamp and pulled longitudinally through the incision
  - ○ The Achillon jig is introduced in the closed position into the paratenon proximally and the arms are progressively widened so that the tendon lays between them (**Fig. 7**)

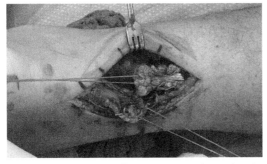

Fig. 5. No. 2 FiberWire is placed in a Krackow suture configuration into each end of the tendon.

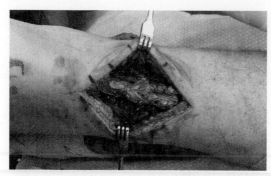

Fig. 6. Tendon ends are reapproximated and secured using a 2-strand construct.

- ○ A needle driver is used to pass the first needle according to the arrows and numbers printed on the jig (**Fig. 8**)
- ○ All 3 sutures are passed sequentially
  - ■ Each suture is marked using a marking pen with 1, 2, or 3 hash marks on each side so that corresponding sutures on each stump may be tied after being pulled out through the incision (**Fig. 9**)
- ○ The Achillon jig is then withdrawn slowly while simultaneously closing the arms of the jig (**Fig. 10**)
  - ■ If any suture fails to grasp the tendon, the above steps must be repeated for that suture only
  - ■ It is important to keep the medial and lateral sutures separate
- ○ The above steps are repeated for the distal tendon stump (**Fig. 11**)
  - ■ Each suture is marked using a marking pen with 1, 2, or 3 hash marks on each side so that, after passing sutures out through the incisions, they can be tied to their corresponding suture limbs on the proximal stump
- ○ The corresponding sutures are then tied while visualizing tendon apposition and maintaining tension similar to the contralateral extremity (**Fig. 12**)
- ○ Close the paratenon with 2-0 Vicryl suture
- ○ Close the subcutaneous tissue with 3-0 Monocryl suture and the skin with 3-0 nylon suture

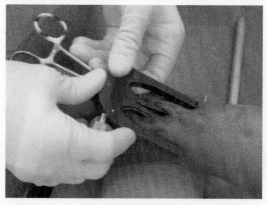

Fig. 7. The Achillon jig is introduced in the closed position into the paratenon proximally and the arms are progressively widened so that the tendon lies between them.

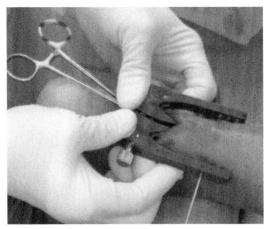

Fig. 8. A needle driver is used to pass the first needle according to the arrows and numbers printed on the jig.

Minimally Invasive Technique Using the Percutaneous Achilles Repair System 3

- Indications:
  - Primary repair of an acute (<3–4 weeks) Achilles tendon rupture occurring between 2 cm and 7 cm above the calcaneal tuberosity
    - Primary repair of tears that are 3 to 6 weeks old may also be performed but require release of scar tissue adhesions between the tendon and paratenon in order to adequately mobilize the tendon ends for apposition
  - Contraindications include chronic ruptures greater than 6 weeks old, prior Achilles surgery, and open ruptures secondary to laceration
- Equipment:
  - PARS system (Arthrex)

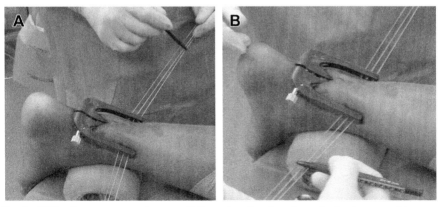

Fig. 9. All 3 sutures are passed sequentially and each suture is marked using a marking pen with 1, 2, or 3 hash marks on each side (*A*, *B*) so that corresponding sutures on each stump may be tied after being pulled out through the incision.

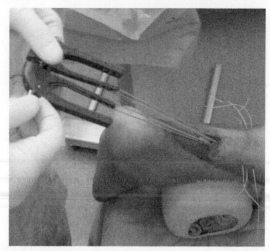

Fig. 10. The Achillon jig is then withdrawn slowly while simultaneously closing the arms of the jig.

- Positioning:
  - Performed with patient prone under general anesthesia with optional popliteal pain catheter for postoperative analgesia
  - Thigh tourniquet placed
  - (Optional) can drape out both legs to compare resting tension of contralateral Achilles tendon

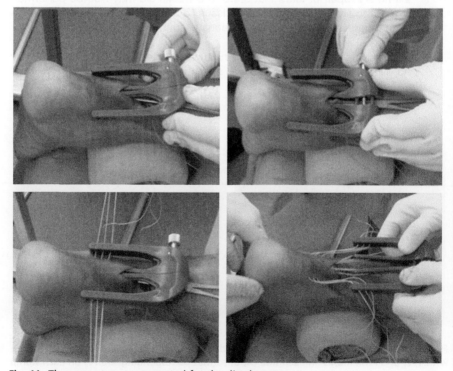

Fig. 11. The same steps are repeated for the distal stump.

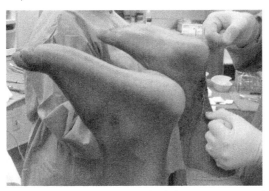

Fig. 12. The corresponding sutures are then tied while visualizing tendon apposition and maintaining tension similar to the contralateral extremity.

- Surgical approach:
  - Transverse 2.5-cm incision is made centrally 1 cm above the palpable Achilles tendon defect (**Fig. 13**)
    - The transverse incision may be extended proximally or distally in a Z-shaped fashion if needed
    - Alternatively, a 2-cm longitudinal incision may be made by starting at the level of the Achilles rupture and traveling 2 cm proximally
  - The paratenon is incised and a finger is used to bluntly palpate the proximal tendon stump as well as release any adhesions

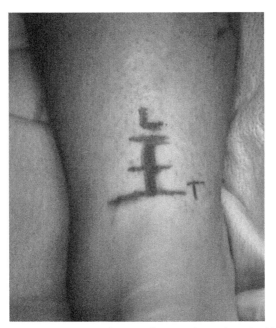

Fig. 13. Transverse 2.5-cm incision is made centrally 1 cm above the palpable Achilles tendon (marked T). Alternatively, a 2-cm longitudinal incision may be made by starting at the level of the Achilles rupture and traveling 2 cm proximally (marked L).

- The proximal stump is grasped with an Allis clamp and pulled longitudinally through the incision
- The PARS jig is then inserted into the proximal paratenon sheath with each arm opened while advancing the jig alongside the proximal Achilles tendon stump (**Fig. 14**)
- A suture-passing needle is inserted through hole 1 and left in place
  - Push down gently on the Achilles tendon to ensure the tendon is captured with each suture needle pass
- A second suture needle is inserted through hole 2 and left in place (see **Fig. 14**)
  - Tension on the proximal stump is maintained by not passing each suture until a second suture-passing needle is in place
- Pass white no. 2 suture via the needle in hole 1 (**Fig. 15**)
- Pass suture needle through oblique hole 3 (see **Fig. 15**)
- Pass blue no. 2 suture via the needle in hole 2 (**Fig. 16**)
- Pass suture needle through oblique hole 4 (see **Fig. 16**)
- Pass nonlooped end of white/green no. 2 suture via the needle in hole 3 (**Fig. 17**)
- Pass suture needle through oblique hole 5 (see **Fig. 17**)
- Pass looped end of white/green no. 2 suture via the needle in hole 4 (**Fig. 18**)
- Pass white/black no. 2 suture via needle in hole 5 (see **Fig. 18**)
  - Optionally, sutures may be passed through holes 6 and 7 if a second locked suture is desired for additional strength

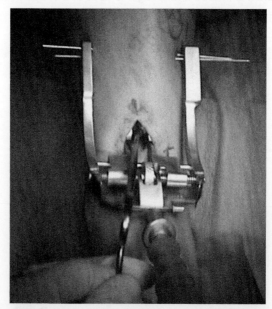

Fig. 14. The paratenon is incised and finger or freer is used to bluntly palpate the proximal tendon stump as well as release any adhesions. The proximal stump is grasped with an Allis clamp and pulled longitudinally to the incision. A PARS jig is then inserted into the proximal paratenon sheath with each arm opened while advancing the jig alongside the proximal Achilles tendon stump. Suture-passing needle is inserted through hole 1 and left in place followed by a second suture needle inserted through hole 2.

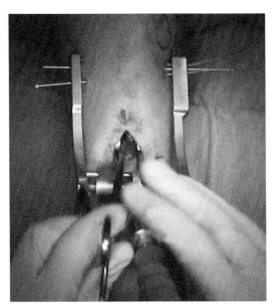

Fig. 15. The white no. 2 FiberWire suture is passed via the needle in hole 1. The suture needle is then passed through oblique hole 3.

- Retract the PARS jig to pull sutures out of the transverse incision (**Fig. 19**)
- Organize the sutures in the same order they were inserted into the jig
- On 1 side, hold both white/green sutures in 1 hand and loop blue suture around the 2 white/green sutures twice, then pass end of blue suture through the looped end of the white green suture (**Fig. 20**)

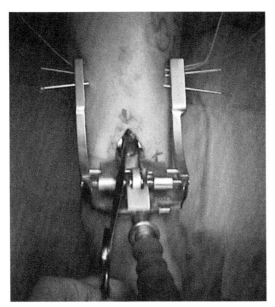

Fig. 16. Blue no. 2 suture is passed via the needle in hole 2. Suture needle is passed through oblique hole 4.

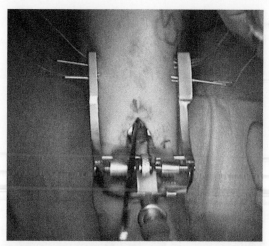

Fig. 17. Nonlooped end of white/green no. 2 suture is passed via the needle in hole 3. Suture needle is then passed through oblique hole 5.

- ○ Repeat for the opposite side
- ○ Pull the unlooped white/green suture end on each side one by one to lock each blue suture (**Fig. 21**)
  - ■ Make sure the 2 blue suture does not fall out of the loop as it is being pulled through
- ○ Pull on the blue suture to ensure that the suture is locked and to minimize creep
- ○ Pull on the white and white/black sutures to ensure that they captured the tendon
  - ■ If any suture missed the tendon, the jig can be reinserted and the suture repassed
- ○ Repeat the above steps for the distal tendon stump
- ○ With the foot slightly plantar flexed, first tie the white/black suture on 1 side of tendon to set tension with Achilles tendon ends opposed while assistant holds limbs of other side to prevent suture from unloading

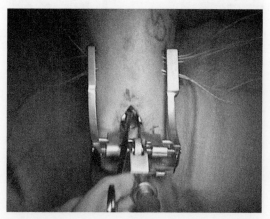

Fig. 18. Looped end of white/green no. 2 suture is passed via the needle in hole 4. White/black no. 2 suture is passed via needle in hole 5.

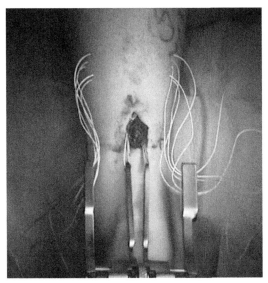

Fig. 19. The PARS jig is retracted to deliver sutures out of the transverse incision.

- Next tie the other side of the white/black suture
- Tie the blue suture on both sides of the Achilles tendon
- Tie the white suture on both sides of the Achilles tendon
- Close the paratenon with 2-0 Vicryl suture
- Close the subcutaneous tissue with 3-0 Monocryl suture and the skin with 3-0 nylon suture

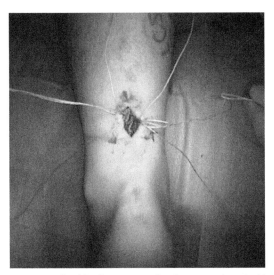

Fig. 20. The sutures are organized in the same order they were inserted into the jig. On one side, both white and green sutures are held in one hand while the blue suture is looped around the 2 white/green sutures twice. The end of the blue suture is then passed through the looped end of the white/green suture. This process is repeated for the opposite side.

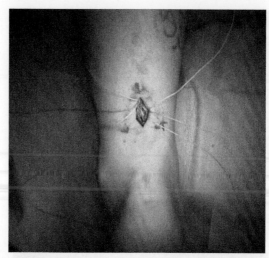

Fig. 21. The unlooped white/green suture end is pulled through on each side one by one to lock each blue suture. The white/green suture is then discarded. The blue suture is then pulled to ensure that the suture is locked and to minimize creep. In addition, the white and white/black sutures are pulled to ensure that they captured the tendon.

Minimally Invasive Technique Using the Internal Brace for Midsubstance Achilles Ruptures (Arthrex Achilles Midsubstance SpeedBridge)

- Indications[20]:
  - Primary repair of an acute (<3 weeks) Achilles tendon rupture occurring between 1 cm and 7 cm above the calcaneal tuberosity
    - Primary repair of tears that are 3 to 6 weeks old may also be performed but require release of scar tissue adhesions between the tendon and paratenon in order to adequately mobilize the tendon ends for apposition
  - This technique has the theoretic advantages of earlier weight bearing, is knotless, and allows direct fixation of the proximal stump to bone
  - Contraindications include chronic ruptures greater than 6 weeks old, prior Achilles surgery, and open ruptures secondary to laceration
- Equipment:
  - PARS instrument and suture kits (Arthrex)
  - Two 4.75-mm Bio-SwiveLock anchors (Arthrex)
  - Suture lasso (Arthrex)
- Positioning:
  - Performed with patient prone under general anesthesia with optional popliteal pain catheter for postoperative analgesia
  - Thigh tourniquet placed
  - (Optional) can drape out both legs to compare resting tension of contralateral Achilles tendon
- Surgical approach:
  - The PARS technique is used to secure the proximal stump of the tendon as previously described (see **Figs. 13–21**); a transverse or longitudinal incision is used 1 cm above the level of the palpable defect
  - Two 0.5-cm to 1-cm longitudinal incisions are made on the posterior aspect of the heel, just below the convex surface of the posterior calcaneus 1 cm away from the midline medially and laterally (**Fig. 22**)

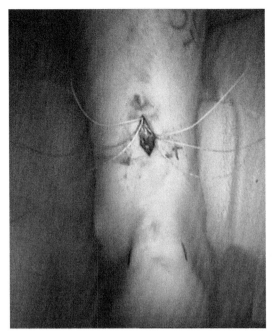

Fig. 22. Two 0.5-cm to 1-cm longitudinal incisions are made on the posterior aspect of the heel, just below the convex surface of the posterior calcaneus 1 cm away from the midline medially and laterally.

- A 3.4-mm drill hole is made in each incision with the drill angled distally and toward the midline (**Fig. 23**)
- The holes are then tapped 2 to 3 times for a 4.75-mm Bio-SwiveLock anchor to ensure the anchor will advance easily (**Fig. 24**)

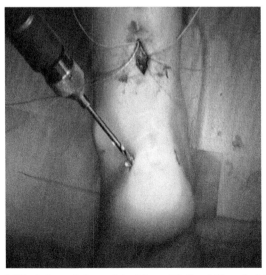

Fig. 23. A 3.4-mm drill hole is made in each incision with the drill angled distally and toward the midline.

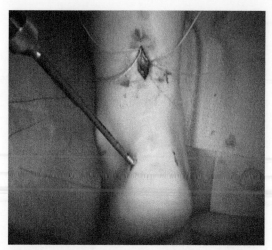

Fig. 24. The holes are then tapped 2 to 3 times for a 4.75-mm Bio-SwiveLock anchor to ensure that the anchor will advance easily.

○ The tip of the Banana SutureLasso (Arthrex) is passed retrograde through each distal incision in the central portion of the distal Achilles tendon stump (**Fig. 25**)
  ■ Ensure that the nitinol wire loop is advanced just short of the tip of the lasso before passing through the tendon
○ Advance the nitinol wire loop and pass the same-side proximal stump sutures through the loop
○ Deliver the proximal sutures through the distal incision by pulling on the Banana SutureLasso and the nitinol wire simultaneously (**Fig. 26**)
○ Repeat for the other side
○ Maximum tension is then placed on the sutures through the distal incision for 10 cycles to diminish creep of the suture
○ The sutures are then passed through the eyelet of the Bio-SwiveLock anchor on each side (**Fig. 27**)
○ The ankle is plantar flexed to oppose the tendon ends
○ With an assistant pulling the opposite-side sutures to set the tension, the anchor is inserted with the suture eyelet advanced to the level of the drill hole (**Fig. 28**)
○ Insert the opposite-side anchor
○ The paratenon is closed with 2-0 Vicryl suture
○ The subcutaneous tissue is closed with 3-0 Monocryl suture and the skin is closed with 3-0 nylon suture (**Fig. 29**)

Rehabilitation Protocol for Acute Achilles Primary Repair (All Techniques)

- The patient is placed a plantar flexed short-leg splint for 2 weeks to allow wound healing
- At 2 weeks, the sutures are removed and a tall boot with 2 peel-away heel lifts is placed
  ○ Alternatively a weight-bearing cast plantar flexed at 10° may be placed
- Physical therapy is initiated at 2 to 4 weeks for ankle range of motion and continued for 8 to 10 weeks

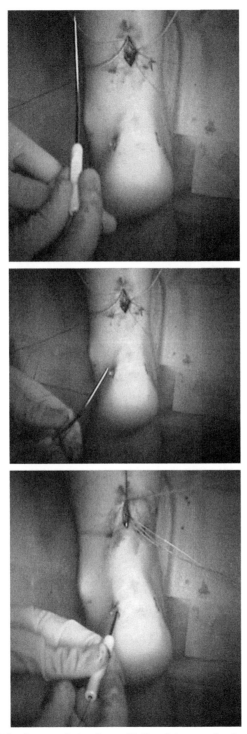

Fig. 25. The tip of the Banana SutureLasso (Arthrex) is passed retrograde through each distal incision in the central portion of the distal Achilles tendon stump. The nitinol wire loop is advanced and the same-side proximal stump sutures are passed through the loop.

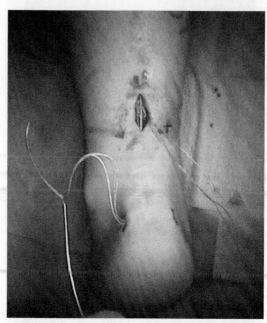

Fig. 26. The proximal sutures are delivered through the distal incision by pulling on the Banana SutureLasso and the nitinol wire simultaneously.

- Formal touch-down (25%) weight bearing with crutches is allowed at 3 weeks with instructions to advance 25% of weight weekly up to full weight bearing and peel away 1 layer of the heel lift each week
  - Weight bearing in the boot with 2 heel lifts may be initiated 1 week after midsubstance internal brace repair
- Patient is transitioned from the boot to regular shoe wear at 8 to 10 weeks
- Nonexplosive activities, including jogging, are advanced beginning at 3 months postoperatively
- Patient is released to full activity at 6 months postoperatively

SURGICAL TREATMENT OPTIONS FOR ACUTE ACHILLES TENDON INSERTIONAL SLEEVE AVULSION
Open Two-suture Anchor Technique

- Indications:
  - Primary repair of an acute (<6 weeks) Achilles tendon insertional sleeve avulsion
  - Presence of Haglund deformity
- Equipment:
  - Two double-loaded suture anchors of choice
  - Fan blade
  - Power rasp
  - Mini C-arm fluoroscopy (optional)
- Positioning:
  - Performed with patient prone under general anesthesia with optional popliteal pain catheter for postoperative analgesia
  - Thigh tourniquet placed

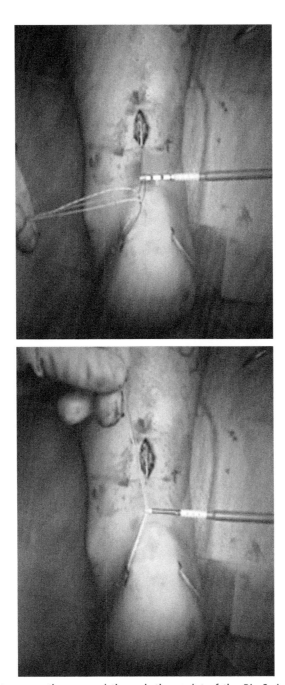

Fig. 27. The sutures are then passed through the eyelet of the Bio-SwiveLock anchor on each side.

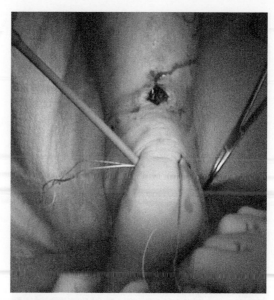

Fig. 28. With an assistant pulling the opposite-side sutures to set the tension, the anchor is inserted with the suture eyelet advanced to the level of the drill hole.

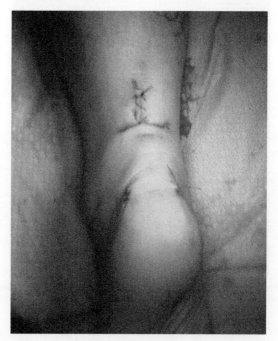

Fig. 29. The paratenon is closed with 2-0 Vicryl suture. The subcutaneous tissue is closed with 3-0 Monocryl suture and the skin is closed with 3-0 nylon suture.

- o (Optional) can drape out both legs to compare resting tension of contralateral Achilles tendon
- Surgical approach:
  - o Longitudinal midline incision is made from 2 to 3 cm above posterosuperior tip of the calcaneal tuberosity to just distal to Achilles tendon
  - o Incise and elevate paratenon layer
  - o Expose Achilles tendon insertion medially and laterally
    - May cut through midline of Achilles tendon from 2 cm above insertion through distal insertion if needed to exposed Haglund deformity
  - o Use fan blade to excise Haglund deformity from posteroinferior to anterosuperior
    - Avoid angling into the subtalar joint
  - o May use power rasp to remove any sharp edges or remaining prominences on medial, lateral, proximal, and distal sides of calcaneal cut
    - Optionally, may confirm adequate Haglund excision under fluoroscopy
  - o Confirm that Achilles tendon stump can be reapproximated to the calcaneal tuberosity with plantar flexion of the foot
    - If unable to reapproximate the Achilles tendon stump, a gastrocnemius recession via a separate central proximal incision may be performed to increase distal tendon stump excursion
    - If Achilles tendon insertion is not repairable or significant diseased tendon present, can augment repair with a flexor hallucis longus (FHL) transfer
  - o Place 2 suture anchors, 1 medially and 1 laterally in distal area of cut calcaneal bone surface 1.5 to 2 cm apart
  - o Pass both limbs of first suture from medial anchor through medial distal Achilles flap 1.5 cm from distal end of tendon and 1 cm apart transversely in tendon flap
  - o Repeat for second anchor laterally
  - o While holding tension on the first suture from one flap, tie the first suture from the other flap
  - o Tie the second suture from the remaining flap
  - o Additional techniques can be used to close the central tendon split using the tails of the sutures from the anchors or additional suture
  - o The paratenon is closed with 2-0 Vicryl suture
  - o The subcutaneous tissue is closed with 3-0 Monocryl suture and the skin is closed with 3-0 nylon suture

Open SpeedBridge Technique

- Indications:
  - o Primary repair of an acute (<6 weeks) Achilles tendon insertional sleeve avulsion
  - o Presence of Haglund deformity
- Equipment:
  - o SpeedBridge set (Arthrex)
  - o Fan blade
  - o Power rasp
  - o Mini C-arm fluoroscopy (optional)
- Positioning:
  - o Performed with patient prone under general anesthesia with optional popliteal pain catheter for postoperative analgesia
  - o Thigh tourniquet placed

- ○ (Optional) can drape out both legs to compare resting tension of contralateral Achilles tendon
- Surgical approach:
  - ○ Longitudinal midline incision is made from 2 to 3 cm above posterosuperior tip of the calcaneal tuberosity to just distal to Achilles tendon
  - ○ Incise and elevate paratenon layer
  - ○ Expose Achilles tendon insertion medially and laterally
    - ■ May cut through midline of Achilles tendon from 2 cm above insertion through distal insertion if needed to exposed Haglund deformity
  - ○ Use fan blade to excise Haglund deformity from posteroinferior to anterosuperior
    - ■ Avoid angling into the subtalar joint
  - ○ Use power rasp to remove any sharp edges or remaining prominences on medial, lateral, proximal, and distal sides of calcaneal cut
    - ■ Optionally, may confirm adequate Haglund excision under fluoroscopy
  - ○ Confirm that Achilles tendon stump can be reapproximated to the calcaneal tuberosity with plantar flexion of the foot
    - ■ If unable to reapproximate the Achilles tendon stump, a gastrocnemius recession via a separate central proximal incision may be performed to increase distal tendon stump excursion
    - ■ If Achilles tendon insertion is not repairable or significant diseased tendon present, can augment repair with an FHL transfer
  - ○ Mark out, drill, and tap for the 2 FiberTape SwiveLock anchors proximally and 2 SwiveLock anchors distally in the cut area of calcaneal bone
    - ■ Tap 2 to 3 times per drill hole in order to ensure smooth insertion of each anchor
  - ○ Insert FiberTape SwiveLock anchors proximally and discard FiberWire suture from anchor
  - ○ Pass both limbs of each anchor through their respective distal Achilles tendon flaps adjacent to one another with the ankle plantar flexed
  - ○ Push each flap down to bone while pulling on both FiberTape limbs for each flap
  - ○ Pass 1 FiberTape limb from each anchor through each of the eyelets of the distal SwiveLock anchors
  - ○ With the Achilles tendon tension set and the ankle plantar flexed, the FiberTape sutures of the first distal SwiveLock anchor are held upward adjacent to the anchor and marked at the laser line on the anchor, which signifies the amount of suture that will be inserted with the anchor
  - ○ The FiberTape suture is then retracted through the eyelet to the level that was marked and tension is held at that point
  - ○ The anchor is then inserted
  - ○ The other anchor is then inserted in the same fashion
  - ○ The paratenon is closed with 2-0 Vicryl suture
  - ○ The subcutaneous tissue is closed with 3-0 Monocryl suture and the skin is closed with 3-0 nylon suture

Rehabilitation Protocol for Acute Achilles Insertional Sleeve Avulsion Repair

- The patient is placed a plantar flexed short leg splint for 2 weeks to allow wound healing
- At 2 weeks, the sutures are removed and a tall boot with 2 peel-away heel lifts is placed
  - ○ Alternatively a weight-bearing cast plantar flexed at 10° may be placed

- Physical therapy is initiated at 2 to 4 weeks for ankle range of motion and continued for 8 to 10 weeks
- Formal touch-down (25%) weight bearing with crutches is allowed at 3 weeks with instructions to advance 25% of weight weekly up to full weight bearing and peel away 1 layer of the heel lift each week
- Patient is transitioned from the boot to regular shoe wear at 8 to 10 weeks
- Nonexplosive activities, including jogging, are advanced at 3 months postoperatively
- Patient is released to full activity at 6 months postoperatively

Complications of Surgical Achilles Repair

Potential complications after acute Achilles repair include sural nerve injury/paresthesias, delayed wound healing, infection, and Achilles reruptures.

Sural nerve injury may lead to postoperative paresthesias. If a neuroma develops that does not respond to conservative management with medication and desensitization, proximal sural nerve excision is recommended.

Delayed wound healing is the most frequently encountered complication after surgical Achilles repair and may hinder rehabilitation. For superficial small areas of wound dehiscence, wet to dry dressings or Silvadene cream may be used to keep the wound clean as it heals. A larger wound dehiscence can be treated with application of negative pressure wound therapy.

Superficial cellulitis after surgical Achilles repair may be treated with oral antibiotics if caught early and there is no evidence of deep infection. Deep infection after acute Achilles repair is a serious complication that should be treated with surgical irrigation and debridement with intravenous antibiotics if there is evidence of cellulitis, draining purulence, underlying abscess, and/or large dehiscence. All infected tissue should be removed, including the tendon repair site if friable and necrotic. If loss of repair is noticed during irrigation and debridement, rerepair should not be attempted until the infection is cleared; typically after 6 weeks. Rerepair may be attempted later if tendon apposition is possible, with or without the use of a V-Y lengthening of the gastrocnemius-soleus fascia depending on mobility of the tendon ends. FHL tendon transfer may be added to augment the repair if the tendon at the repair site is of poor quality or if tendon apposition is not possible.

Achilles rerupture, although uncommon, typically requires surgical management. Open primary repair is recommended with possible use of V-Y gastrocnemius-soleus fascia lengthening and possible use of FHL tendon transfer depending on the quality of the tendon. If tendon apposition is not possible, then FHL tendon transfer or allograft tendon reconstruction may be considered.

SUMMARY

Achilles tendon rupture is a common lower extremity injury seen in the active population. Although reruptures rates have improved with nonoperative functional management, surgical treatment is still preferred by the authors. Minimally invasive techniques allow optimal Achilles tendon rupture apposition and tensioning, with a reduced risk of soft tissue complications associated with the traditional open repair.

REFERENCES

1. Maffulli N, Waterston SW, Squair J, et al. Changing incidence of Achilles tendon rupture in Scotland: a 15-year study. Clin J Sport Med 1999;9(3):157–60.

2. Houshian S, Tscherning T, Riegels-Nielsen P. The epidemiology of Achilles tendon rupture in a Danish county. Injury 1998;29(9):651–4.

3. Gwynne-Jones DP, Sims M, Handcock D. Epidemiology and outcomes of acute Achilles tendon rupture with operative or nonoperative treatment using an identical functional bracing protocol. Foot Ankle Int 2011;32(4):337–43.

4. Bhandari M, Guyatt GH, Siddiqui F, et al. Treatment of acute Achilles tendon ruptures: a systematic overview and metaanalysis. Clin Orthop Relat Res 2002;(400): 190–200.

5. Willits K, Amendola A, Bryant D, et al. Operative versus nonoperative treatment of acute Achilles tendon ruptures: a multicenter randomized trial using accelerated functional rehabilitation. J Bone Joint Surg Am 2010;92(17):2767–75.

6. Ma GW, Griffith TG. Percutaneous repair of acute closed ruptured Achilles tendon: a new technique. Clin Orthop Relat Res 1977;(128):247–55.

7. Cretnik A, Zlajpah L, Smrkolj V, et al. The strength of percutaneous methods of repair of the Achilles tendon: a biomechanical study. Med Sci Sports Exerc 2000;32(1):16–20.

8. Lim J, Dalal R, Waseem M. Percutaneous vs. open repair of the ruptured Achilles tendon–a prospective randomized controlled study. Foot Ankle Int 2001;22(7): 559–68.

9. Kakiuchi M. A combined open and percutaneous technique for repair of tendo Achillis. Comparison with open repair. J Bone Joint Surg Br 1995;77(1):60–3.

10. Assal M, Jung M, Stern R, et al. Limited open repair of Achilles tendon ruptures: a technique with a new instrument and findings of a prospective multicenter study. J Bone Joint Surg Am 2002;84-A(2):161–70.

11. Hsu AR, Jones CP, Cohen BE, et al. Clinical outcomes and complications of percutaneous Achilles repair system versus open technique for acute Achilles tendon ruptures. Foot Ankle Int 2015;36(11):1279–86.

12. Cretnik A, Kosanovic M, Smrkolj V. Percutaneous versus open repair of the ruptured Achilles tendon: a comparative study. Am J Sports Med 2005;33(9): 1369–79.

13. Ahmad J, Repka M, Raikin SM. Treatment of myotendinous Achilles ruptures. Foot Ankle Int 2013;34(8):1074–8.

14. Huh J, Easley ME, Nunley JA 2nd. Characterization and surgical management of Achilles tendon sleeve avulsions. Foot Ankle Int 2016;37(6):596–604.

15. Maffulli N. The clinical diagnosis of subcutaneous tear of the Achilles tendon. A prospective study in 174 patients. Am J Sports Med 1998;26(2):266–70.

16. Griffin MJ, Olson K, Heckmann N, et al. Realtime Achilles Ultrasound Thompson (RAUT) test for the evaluation and diagnosis of acute Achilles tendon ruptures. Foot Ankle Int 2017;38(1):36–40.

17. Yepes H, Tang M, Geddes C, et al. Digital vascular mapping of the integument about the Achilles tendon. J Bone Joint Surg Am 2010;92(5):1215–20.

18. Jaakkola JI, Hutton WC, Beskin JL, et al. Achilles tendon rupture repair: biomechanical comparison of the triple bundle technique versus the Krakow locking loop technique. Foot Ankle Int 2000;21(1):14–7.

19. Labib SA, Rolf R, Dacus R, et al. The "Giftbox" repair of the Achilles tendon: a modification of the Krackow technique. Foot Ankle Int 2009;30(5):410–4.

20. McWilliam JR, Mackay G. The internal brace for midsubstance Achilles ruptures. Foot Ankle Int 2016;37(7):794–800.

The Missed Achilles Tear
Now what?

Brian D. Steginsky, DO[a,1], Bryan Van Dyke, DO[b,2], Gregory C. Berlet, MD[b,*]

KEYWORDS

- Achilles • Chronic Achilles tendon ruptures • Neglected Achilles tendon ruptures
- Tendon transfer for Achilles ruptures • V-Y advancement

KEY POINTS

- Chronic Achilles tendon ruptures are debilitating injuries and are often associated with large tendon gaps that can be challenging for the foot and ankle surgeon to treat.
- Preoperative evaluation must include the patient's functional goals, medical comorbidities, MRI assessment of gastrocnemius-soleus muscle viability, condition of adjacent flexor tendons, and size of the tendon defect to formulate an individualized treatment plan.
- Several techniques have been described for the surgical management of chronic Achilles tendon ruptures, including V-Y advancement, gastrocnemius turndown flaps, tendon transfers, autograft and allograft, and synthetic material augmentation.
- The authors believe flexor hallucis longus transfer to the calcaneus, performed through a single-incision technique, is critical to restore push-off power. We no longer perform isolated V-Y advancement because of the cosmetically unacceptable scar and need to restore plantar flexion strength.

INTRODUCTION

The treatment of chronic Achilles tendon ruptures presents a unique challenge for foot and ankle surgeons. Often, these present as a missed or neglected injury, adding to the complexity of treating an already debilitating tendon rupture. Several surgical techniques have been described in the treatment of chronic Achilles tendon ruptures. Although the length of the tendon defect is often used to guide surgical decision-making, the authors believe that a comprehensive evaluation and awareness of the various treatment options are also critical to successful patient outcomes. Appropriate preoperative evaluation should include the patient's

---

Disclosure Statement: The authors have nothing to disclose.
[a] Illinois Bone & Joint Institute, 720 Florsheim Drive, Libertyville, IL 60048, USA; [b] The Orthopedic Foot & Ankle Center, 300 Polaris Parkway, Suite 2000, Westerville, OH 43082, USA
[1] 720 Florsheim Drive, Libertyville, IL 60048.
[2] 300 Polaris Parkway, Suite 2000, Westerville, OH 43082.
* Corresponding author.
E-mail address: ofacresearch@orthofootankle.com

functional goals and medical comorbidities, MRI assessment of gastrocnemius-soleus muscle viability, viability of adjacent flexor tendons, and size of tendon defect to formulate an individualized treatment plan for the patient. Surgical management carries the risks of wound complications and potential difficulties in re-establishing a functional musculotendinous unit. This article reviews the principles of diagnosis, treatment options, and clinical outcomes, and outlines the authors' preferred techniques.

DEFINITIONS OF CHRONIC AND NEGLECTED ACHILLES TENDON RUPTURE

Missed, chronic, and neglected are terms that have been used interchangeably to describe Achilles tendon ruptures that have either not been appropriately diagnosed or treated after rupture.[1] It is estimated that 25% of acute Achilles tendon ruptures are missed at the initial office visit.[2] Chronic ruptures are most frequently the product of an unrecognized injury, misdiagnosis, or late patient presentation.[3] Although there are slight discrepancies, many investigators recognize 4 to 6 weeks from the time of injury as a chronic rupture.[3,4] When there is a delay in treatment, the term neglected rupture is often used to describe the injury.[1,4] Synonymous use of these terms results in an overlap of definitions in the literature.

EVALUATION AND DIAGNOSIS

The classic signs and symptoms of an acute Achilles tendon rupture are not always present in the patient with a neglected injury. The pain and swelling associated with an acute rupture, although present to some degree, often dissipate with time. Individuals may report fatigability and loss of strength in the affected calf, particularly involving activities that demand repetitive plantar flexion. The ability to ascend and descend stairs, hike, and run may be severely compromised. The muscles of the deep posterior compartment of the leg preserve the ability to perform some active plantar flexion, potentially concealing a complete Achilles tendon rupture. It is not uncommon for a limp to be present.[3]

The physician should inquire about functional demands and medical comorbidities. Surgical intervention may not be appropriate for low-demand individuals or patients with a history of peripheral vascular disease, diabetes, smoking, or noncompliance.

Observing the patient in the prone position, the contralateral extremity should be used for side-by-side comparison. Visual inspection and circumferential girth measurements may reveal significant muscle atrophy of the leg. Dynamic examination of plantar flexion strength can be evaluated by having the patient walk on their tiptoes and perform a single-heel rise. Fatigue and weakness is more evident with repetitive heel-rise.[1] Gait should be observed for the presence of an antalgic limp or altered kinematics. Fibrous scar may bridge the tendon stumps and a palpable defect may be absent.

Several clinical tests have been described for acute Achilles tendon ruptures but are less sensitive for neglected injuries.[4] The Thompson test is performed by squeezing the calf with the patient in the prone position and observing the plantar flexion of the foot.[5] If there is complete discontinuity in the Achilles tendon, plantar flexion of the foot will be absent. Cuttica and colleagues[6] performed a cadaveric study to determine the sensitivity of the Thompson test after progressive sectioning of the Achilles tendon and deep flexor tendons. The Thompson sign was absent in all specimens after complete sectioning of the Achilles tendon. However, the Thompson sign remained intact after sectioning up to 75% of the Achilles tendon and all the deep flexor tendons. The Thompson test may be falsely intact in a neglected Achilles tendon rupture if interposed scar tissue reestablishes continuity between the ends of the tendon. The Matles test is performed with the patient prone and the knees flexed to 90°.[7] Gravity will drive the foot of the affected extremity into a more dorsiflexed position compared with the uninjured side. The O'Brien test involves placing a needle into the Achilles tendon 10 cm proximal to its insertion.[8] The examiner passively positions the foot into dorsiflexion while observing movement of the needle. If the Achilles tendon is ruptured, the needle will not move during passive dorsiflexion of the foot.

MRI and ultrasound can be used to confirm the diagnosis of a neglected Achilles tendon rupture, evaluate the magnitude of the defect, and assess the status of the gastrocnemius-soleus muscle belly. Ultrasound examination of a normal Achilles tendon will demonstrate a hypoechogenic band with well-defined margins.[4] Changes in signal echogenicity and tendon discontinuity are typically present after an Achilles tendon rupture (**Fig. 1**).[3,4,9] Although ultrasound may provide a rapid and cost-effective approach in the diagnosis of an Achilles tendon rupture, it's sensitivity is highly user-dependent.[9]

MRI should be used to evaluate the gastrocnemius-soleus muscle belly for signs of chronic atrophy, including fat-infiltration and fibrosis (**Fig. 2**). Repair should only be undertaken if the muscle belly is found to be viable on preoperative MRI evaluation. The presence of fibrosis and fatty-infiltration portends an incomplete and unsatisfactory recuperation of muscle function after tendon repair. Tendon transfers, as an adjunct to Achilles repair, should be performed if fibrosis and fatty infiltration is evident on preoperative MRI. Radiographs may be helpful to rule out an avulsion injury of the calcaneus. Preoperative imaging should be used to devise a surgical strategy, keeping in mind that the magnitude of the defect will likely change after intraoperative debridement.

NONOPERATIVE TREATMENT

Chronic or neglected Achilles tendon ruptures can lead to significant pain and functional deficits. With failed diagnosis and treatment, the overall length of the Achilles tendon is increased. This decreases plantarflexion strength, which affects the gait and decreases ankle stability. Neglected Achilles tendon ruptures demonstrate

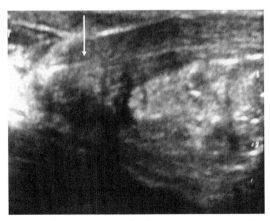

Fig. 1. Ultrasound examination of a chronic Achilles tendon rupture. There is loss of Achilles tendon continuity and conformity. The arrow points to the bulbous distal tendon stump. (*From* Maffulli N, Ajis A. Management of chronic ruptures of the Achilles tendon. J Bone Joint Surg Am 2008;90(6):1350; with permission.)

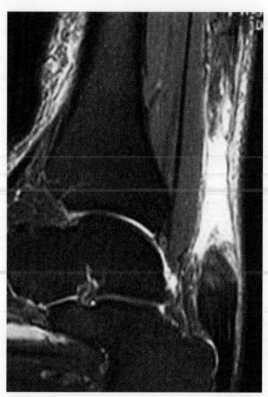

Fig. 2. Sagittal T2 MRI of a chronic Achilles tendon rupture. The high signal intensity correlates with a complete Achilles tendon rupture with a large gap distance. There is fatty infiltration of the proximal gastrocsoleus muscle belly. (*From* Leslie HDH, Edwards WHB. Neglected ruptures of the Achilles tendon. Foot Ankle Clin 2005;10(2):360; with permission.)

approximately 36% of normal plantarflexion strength compared with the unaffected limb.[10] This can lead to decreased stride length, difficulty with stairs, and an inability to run.

Historically, nonoperative management of chronic Achilles tendon ruptures involved immobilization in equinus with serial casting in progressive ankle dorsiflexion. Christensen[11] reported on treatment of 57 Achilles tendon ruptures, with 18 chronic Achilles tendon ruptures treated nonoperatively. Ten (55.6%) of these subjects reported satisfactory results, defined by a normal gait, return to previous occupation, and minimal discomfort. However, they noted that the recovery process was prolonged, often taking several years. Comparatively, 29 (74.3%) out of 39 surgically treated subjects reported satisfactory results. Poor patient satisfaction associated with nonsurgical treatment has led some surgeons to reserve nonoperative management for patients considered high risk for complications.

Nonsurgical management obviates the risks associated with surgery, including wound complications and sural nerve injury. Bruggeman and colleagues[12] reported an overall complication rate of 10.4% in a cohort of 164 subjects undergoing acute Achilles tendon rupture repair. They found independent risk factors to be tobacco use, steroid use, and female sex. The complication rate was 42.1% in subjects with at least 1 risk factor compared with 6.2% in subjects with no identifiable risk factors. The risk of deep vein thrombosis (DVT) has been proposed to be increased in subjects treated surgically for chronic Achilles ruptures compared with acute ruptures.[13] This study did not compare surgical and nonsurgical treatment. Three (17.6%) DVTs and 2 (11.8%) pulmonary emboli were reported in the cohort of 17 surgically treated subjects with chronic Achilles ruptures. They suggested that the DVTs may have developed before surgery and were attributed to immobility despite the subjects being weightbearing preoperatively. They recommend chemical DVT prophylaxis in all surgically treated chronic Achilles ruptures. DVT should be considered a risk for both operatively and nonoperatively treated Achilles ruptures.

More recent advancements in functional rehabilitation protocols have improved nonsurgical outcome.[14] Functional rehabilitation protocols typically begin with 2 weeks of immobilization in plantarflexion. After 2 weeks, plantarflexion-resistance exercises are initiated with the patient fitted into an orthosis that prevents dorsiflexion. The degree of dorsiflexion allowed is progressively advanced each week. However, most of these favorable studies have involved only acute Achilles tendon ruptures. To date, there is no literature demonstrating similar functional outcomes with nonoperative functional rehabilitation protocols for chronic or neglected Achilles tendon ruptures.

SURGICAL TREATMENT ALGORITHMS FOR CHRONIC RUPTURES

There is a paucity of literature comparing the various methods of repair for chronic and neglected Achilles tendon ruptures. Treatment algorithms are based on level 5 evidence (expert opinion).[1,15,16] The size of the tendon defect remains the foundation for most investigators' treatment recommendations. The authors review the literature on published techniques and outline our preferred approaches to the chronic Achilles tendon tear.

DIRECT END-TO-END REPAIR

The large gap distance associated with neglected Achilles tendon ruptures make apposition of the tendon ends challenging and often impedes the ability to perform a direct end-to-end repair. The tendon stumps retract within the paratenon, disorganized fibrovascular scar tissue fills the void, and the myotendinous unit heals in an elongated, weaker state (**Fig. 3**).[4] Debridement of the interposed scar tissue enlarges the size of the defect (**Fig. 4**). The ability to perform an end-to-end repair is limited by retraction of the proximal tendon end, magnitude of the defect after debridement, and tendon excursion after lysis of adhesions. Using end-to-end anastomosis for chronic ruptures with defects, postdebridement of less than 2 cm can be achieved.[1] Tension applied to the proximal tendon stump for several minutes, along with release of scar adhesions ventrally, permits stress relaxation of the myotendinous junction and can provide up to 2 cm in length. The authors recommend end-to-end repair only when the continuity of the tendon can be re-established without excessive plantarflexion of the foot or undue tension at the site of anastomosis. Maximal plantarflexion to facilitate a direct end-to-end repair is unlikely to maintain continuity. If plantar flexion greater than 30° is required for end-to-end anastomosis, we recommend a proximal lengthening technique (gastrocsoleus lengthening or V-Y lengthening) to re-establish the continuity but a flexor tendon transfer for the re-establishment of plantar flexion power.

Another technique to bridge a large gap is to limit debridement of the interposed scar tissue and use some of this tissue to assist in tendon stump apposition and direct end-to-end repair.[17,18] Successful end-to-end repair with incorporation of scar tissue

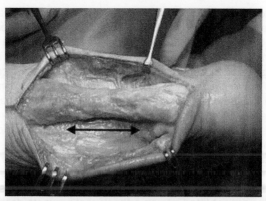

Fig. 3. Interposed fibrous scar tissue bridges the tendon ends in a chronic Achilles tendon rupture. The double arrow demonstrates the region of elongated scar tissue. (*From* Yasuda T, Shima H, Mori K, et al. Direct repair of chronic achilles tendon ruptures using scar tissue located between the tendon stumps. J Bone Joint Surg Am 2016;98(14);1170; with permission.)

has been achieved in neglected Achilles tendon ruptures with defects up to 5 cm.[17] Porter and colleagues[17] were the first to report on the functional outcomes after end-to-end repair using interposed scar tissue for neglected Achilles tendon ruptures. Eleven subjects underwent end-to-end repair at an average of 47 days from the time of injury. The tendon stumps were freshened and circumferential lysis of adhesions was performed to facilitate stump excursion. The interposed fibrous scar tissue was then used to imbricate the tendon stumps. Incorporation of the scar tissue facilitated stump apposition without the need for a fascial advancement or gastrocnemius turndown flap. Defects ranged from 3 to 5 cm before mobilization of the tendon ends. At a minimum of 18-months follow-up, all subjects had excellent functional outcomes and no reruptures were reported.

It has been often discussed that the interposed soft tissue is inadequate in strength and the repetitive cyclic loading of the interposed scar tissue results in elongation of

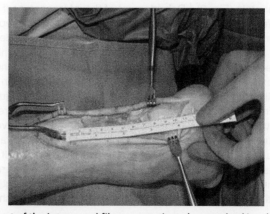

Fig. 4. Debridement of the interposed fibrous scar tissue has resulted in a large gap distance. (*From* Ofili KP, Pollard JD, Schuberth JM. The neglected achilles tendon rupture repaired with allograft: a retrospective review of 14 cases. J Foot Ankle Surg 2016;55(6):1246; with permission.)

the myotendinous unit.[19] On the contrary, histologic examination of the interposed scar tissue after neglected Achilles tendon rupture reveals myxoid stroma, collagen fascicles, and an abundance of fibrovascular granulation tissue suggestive of its reparative potential.[17] Other investigators have shown that histologic evaluation of the interposed scar tissue at the time of surgery reveals a dense collagen network with occasional fibers oriented parallel to the longitudinal axis of the Achilles tendon, a highly cellular vascular stroma, and no evidence of mucoid degeneration.[18] Yasuda and colleagues[18] reported on 30 subjects with neglected or misdiagnosed Achilles tendon ruptures who underwent end-to-end repair with incorporation of the scar tissue at an average of 22 weeks from injury. Postoperative improvements in the American Orthopaedic Foot and Ankle Society (AOFAS) ankle-hindfoot score, ankle range of motion, calf circumference, return to activity, and ability to perform a single-leg heel rise were reported at an average of 33-months follow-up. There were no reruptures and only a single wound complication was reported.

The authors advocate direct end-to end-repair when the postdebridement gap is less than 2 cm and the repair can be achieved with a plantar flexion less than 30°.

V-Y TENDO-ACHILLES ADVANCEMENT

Tendon defects of 2 to 5 cm can be treated with V-Y advancement. V-Y lengthening technique is done at the level of the fascia proximally with the goal of avoiding a cut into the muscle. The rule of thumb for the inverted V fascia cut is that the arms of the V cut should be 1.5 times the measured defect distally. This allows an arithmetical approach to planning the arms of the V-Y. The problem with the V-Y is that it is a large and often cosmetically poor surgical scar. The other challenge is that fascial advancement procedures, including V-Y lengthening and gastrocnemius turndown flaps, lengthen the myotendinous unit, resulting in nonphysiologic resting tension of the sarcomeres and weakness with plantar flexion.[17]

We make a distal longitudinal incision placed medially to the Achilles tendon. As the incision is extended proximally, the incision is curved directly over the posterior midline of the calf. Care should be taken to preserve the sural nerve and paratenon (for later repair). The fibrous pseudotendon is debrided to healthy tendon edges. The gap distance is measured with the knee in approximately 30° of flexion and the ankle in 20° of plantarflexion. An inverted V-incision is made only through the tendinous portion of the gastrocsoleus complex. The apex of the inverted-V should be placed at the most proximal aspect of the myotendinous junction. The limbs of the inverted-V should be at least 1.5 times the length of the measured defect and exit at the medial and lateral boarders of the tendon. Care is taken to minimize the amount of muscle undermining, although tendon excursion can sometimes be limited by the underlying muscle belly fibers. The inverted-Y is repaired in a side-to-side fashion using a number 2 nonabsorbable suture (**Fig. 5**).

Abraham and Pankovich[20] were the first to describe the surgical technique of V-Y advancement in 4 subjects who underwent repair for chronic Achilles tendon rupture. Defects up to 5 to 6 cm were repaired with V-Y gastrocnemius recession followed by suture repair of the tendon ends. They report a return of calf strength and ability to perform a single leg heel-rise in 3 subjects, although 1 subject continued to demonstrate weakness and an inability to perform a single leg heel-rise. The only complication was sural neuroma. V-Y advancement has been successfully reported in the repair of chronic Achilles tendon ruptures with defects exceeding 10 cm.[21] Myerson[1] recommends V-Y advancement alone for defects that are less than 5 cm.

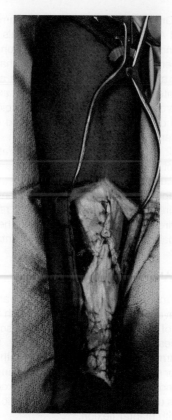

Fig. 5. V-Y advancement for chronic Achilles tendon rupture.

Parker and Repinecz[22] described a modification of the original V-Y advancement that involves a tongue-in-groove gastrocnemius recession. They state that the tongue-in-groove recession is easier to perform than V-Y advancement and provides up to 50% more length. The tongue-in-groove technique was described in a single case report and is less commonly used to treat neglected Achilles tendon ruptures than V-Y advancement.

Plantar flexion weakness is uniformly present after V-Y advancement for chronic Achilles tendon ruptures.[23–25] Kissel and colleagues[24] reported up to a 30% deficit in plantar flexion peak torque after V-Y advancement compared with the uninjured extremity. Elias and colleagues[23] reported on 15 subjects with missed or neglected Achilles tendon ruptures who had V-Y advancement augmented with flexor hallucis longus (FHL) tendon transfer. At mean follow-up of 2 years, all subjects were reportedly satisfied with their outcome, despite an average plantar flexion peak torque deficit ranging from 13.5% to 22.3% after repair. The loss of plantar flexion strength after fascia advancement procedures is permanent. Guclu and colleagues[26] reported an average plantar flexion peak torque deficit of 16% (30° per second) and 17% (120° per second) in 17 subjects who had V-Y advancement with fascia-flap turndown for chronic Achilles tendon rupture at 16-years follow-up. The mean AOFAS ankle-hindfoot score at last follow-up was 95 out of 100, paralleling the scores previous reported by Elias and colleagues.[23] The permanent loss of calf strength after V-Y advancement does not seem to have a negative effect on patient satisfaction and functional outcomes at both short-term and long-term follow-up.

The authors rarely use the V-Y lengthening due to the cosmetically unacceptable scar and the need for flexor tendon augmentation to restore push-off power. We believe that other techniques allow bridging of the gap distally and we rely on the flexor tendon transfer of the FHL for functional and strength improvements.

GASTROCNEMIUS TURNDOWN FLAPS

The Strayer gastrocnemius recession was first described to treat calf spasticity in cerebral palsy subjects but has since been extrapolated to the treatment of neglected Achilles tendon ruptures to help reestablish continuity without undue tension at the repair.[27,28]

Several investigators have used the gastrocnemius fascia turndown flap to span the large defect associated with neglected Achilles tendon ruptures.[12,19,29,30] Fascia turndown flaps have also been used to augment direct end-to-end repairs with V-Y advancement to strengthen the repair site.[25,26,31,32]

Christensen[11] elevated a 2-cm by 10-cm flap from the proximal gastrocnemius fascia and turned the flap downward to span the tendon defect. The flap was anastomosed to the distal tendon segment. The pedicle of the turndown flap was reinforced with suture to prevent complete avulsion. The defect in the proximal tendon segment was closed in a side-to-side fashion. Christensen[11] reported the return to work, normal gait, and only slight discomfort in 75% (25/33) of subjects after performing a fascia turndown flap for acute or neglected Achilles tendon ruptures. Silverskiold[33] described a similar technique to Christensen,[11] although the flap was rotated 180° to orient the smooth surface posteriorly.

Lindholm[34] developed a technique to avoid injury to the arteries located in the midline of the aponeurosis and to minimize scar adhesions. He cut a 1-cm by 8-cm flap on either side of the gastrocnemius aponeurosis located approximately 1 cm from the midline. The flaps were twisted backwards such that the smooth serosal surface faced posteriorly and were sutured to the proximal and distal Achilles tendon segments. Arner and Lindholm[29] reported on 86 subjects with acute or neglected Achilles tendon ruptures who underwent 1 of 4 different methods of repair: end-to-end anastomosis (20), Silverskiold (25), Christensen (30), and Lindholm technique (11). Excellent or good results were reported 79 out of 82 subjects available for follow-up. There was no difference in functional outcomes between the various techniques, although the Lindholm technique was the only method that was not associated with tethering and adhesions at the repair site.

Takao and colleagues[35] reported on 10 subjects with neglected Achilles tendon ruptures who were treated with the Lindholm technique. Excellent functional outcomes were reported, despite plantar flexion peak torque deficits up to 23% in the operative extremity. The mean AOFAS score at an average follow-up of 6 years was 98.1 plus or minus 2.5. No reruptures were reported.

Bosworth[19] used a 0.5-inch by 9-inch fascia turndown flap that was woven transversely through the proximal and distal tendon segments and secured back onto itself with suture. No complications or reruptures were reported in the cohort of 6 subjects with neglected Achilles tendon ruptures. Lee and colleagues[36] reported good-to-excellent outcomes using the Leppilahti scoring system in 11 out of 12 subjects with neglected Achilles tendon ruptures after a modified Bosworth technique.

Rush[30] developed a gastrocnemius aponeurosis flap that was tubularized by suturing the margins together. The distal tendon segment was placed into the tabularized flap and an anastomosis was performed. All 5 subjects included in the study were reportedly happy with the results at follow-up.

Cadaveric studies demonstrate greater ultimate tensile strength with fascia turndown augmentation over simple end-to-end repair.[37] Gerdes and colleagues[37] determined the ultimate load to failure after fascia turndown augmentation was 217.5 N compared with 153.9 N after simple end-to-end repair. Although fascia augmentation of an Achilles tendon rupture may improve the mechanical strength of the repair, recent literature has challenged its functional benefits.

Pajala and colleagues[38] reported on 60 subjects with Achilles tendon ruptures that were randomized into 2 groups: simple end-to-end repair or augmented repair as described by Silfverskiold.[33] There were no differences in outcomes between the 2 groups at 12 months follow up. Fascia augmentation was associated with an increase in operative time by a mean of 25 minutes and required a longer skin incision compared with simple end-to-end repair. Tendon elongation and loss of strength was documented in both groups. Heikkinen and colleagues[39] also found no benefit after fascia augmentation over simple end-to-end repair at 14-years follow-up. There is paucity in the literature to advocate for the superiority of any single technique or the routine use of augmentation. Similar to V-Y advancement, cosmetically displeasing extensile incisions are necessary to harvest a proximal turndown flap. Additionally, the soft-tissue disruption associated with the extensile incision and longer surgical time can lead to increased scar formation, adhesions, and higher rates of wound complications.

Although the turndown flap fails to restore adequate plantarflexion strength when performed alone, when performed in conjunction with FHL tendon transfer, it restores the natural contour of the Achilles tendon. The authors have found that restoring the natural contour of the hindfoot permits unimpeded footwear and improved patient satisfaction. The FHL tendon transfer provides a viable myotendinous unit, capable of hypertrophy, and subsequent restoration of plantarflexion power.

GAP BRIDGING USING AUTOGENOUS AND NONAUTOGENOUS SOURCES

Alternatives to bridge the gap of a chronic Achilles tear are autograft fascia lata grafts, interposition allograft tendon or patches, xenograft patches, or synthetic lattices.

Tendon Allograft

Achilles tendon allograft has been used to bridge defects up to 12 cm in neglected Achilles tendon ruptures with good patient outcomes.[40–45] Nellas and colleagues[44] first reported the use of an Achilles tendon allograft for 4.5-cm tendon defect after a failed primary repair secondary to infection. Two strips of freeze-dried Achilles tendon allograft were superimposed on each other, sutured to the proximal and distal Achilles tendon stumps, and augmented with a pull-out suture.

Hanna and colleagues[41] used Achilles tendon allograft with bone block fixation in 6 subjects with chronic Achilles tendon ruptures or severe tendinosis. The diseased portion of the Achilles tendon and its insertion onto the calcaneal tuberosity were excised, allowing bone block allograft fixation to the calcaneus with 2 4.5-mm cannulated screws. The foot was placed in plantar flexion to appropriately tension the repair and anastomosed to the proximal tendon stump. All subjects were satisfied with the procedure and no reruptures were reported. Despite the potential advantages of bone-to-bone healing, bone block allograft has been associated with delayed union in small case reports.[45]

The replacement of the diseased or chronically torn Achilles tendon using allograft tendon, with or without anchoring to the calcaneus, is considered experimental and is supported by only weak-level evidence in the published literature. There are some patient circumstances that may make Achilles tendon allograft more suitable, such as large tendon gaps greater than 10 cm or patients in whom tendon transfer is not an option.[46] Cienfuegos and colleagues[40] published a case report on a chronic Achilles rupture with a 12-cm defect treated with a fresh Achilles tendon allograft. The patient was a 43-year-old male construction worker and was reported to return to normal activities at 1 year. The surgeon and patient must also consider that the use of allograft tissue carries a risk, though low, of disease transmission and increased cost.

Autograft Augmentation

Fascia lata autograft has been used to reconstruct the tendon defect associated with chronic Achilles tendon ruptures with acceptable patient outcomes.[47,48] Bugg and Boyd[49] reported on 10 subjects with neglected Achilles tendon ruptures that were repaired using 3 strips of fascia lata harvested from the proximal thigh. The strips were sutured to the proximal and distal tendon segments, then subsequently over-wrapped using a tubularized-sheet of fascia lata with the serosal side facing outwards. Pull-out suture was used to augment the repair. They reported "satisfactory functional and cosmetic results and no difficulty with adherent scars."[49]

More recent literature has demonstrated the utility of a composite anterolateral thigh free flap with vascularized fascia lata to reconstruct Achilles tendon defects with associated with overlying soft-tissue loss.[50,51] Duhamel and colleagues[50] reported on a subject who developed a postoperative hematoma and subsequent overlying skin necrosis after revision Achilles tendon repair. Satisfactory tendon healing was reported at 1-year follow-up on clinical and MRI examination after the tendon defect and overlying skin necrosis was treated with an anterolateral thigh free flap with vascularized fascia lata.

Maffulli and Leadbetter[52] used gracilis tendon autograft to repair Achilles tendon defects in 21 subjects with neglected Achilles tendon ruptures. The average gap distance was 6.8 cm, but deficits up to 9 cm were successfully repaired using this technique. The gracilis tendon harvest was performed through a separate incision over the pes anserinus, and the graft was woven transversely through the distal and proximal tendon segments. Five subjects developed a superficial wound infection but did not require any further surgical intervention. Three subjects reported hypersensitivity or developed a hypertrophic scar at the surgical incision. Fifteen subjects were available for follow-up at a mean of 10.9 years after surgery.[53] Most subjects reported excellent or good outcomes with minimal limitations, despite permanent loss of strength as reflected by a mean peak torque deficit of 73.1 N in the operative extremity. Only 2 subjects reported fair results with mild to moderate pain, persistent limitations with recreational and daily activities, moderate footwear restrictions, and major reservations with surgery.

Semitendinosus tendon autograft has also been used to successfully reconstruct large defects in chronic Achilles tendon ruptures. Dumbre and colleagues[54] passed semitendinosus tendon autograft through a tunnel in the calcaneus, securing the autograft back onto itself, before performing an anastomosis with the proximal tendon segment. They reported satisfactory functional outcomes, good soft tissue healing, and no reruptures.

The authors do not use autogenous sourced grafts for the bridging of chronic Achilles defects. The harvest site morbidity, the negative influence on our ability to use regional anesthesia, and the availability of excellent alternatives without these challenges has made these autogenous sourced grafts not useful in our practice.

Synthetics

Synthetic materials avoid donor site morbidity and minimize operative time associated with autograft harvest. Unlike allografts, synthetic materials do not carry the risk of disease transmission. However, synthetic materials have been postulated to be associated with a higher risk of wound complications, infection, and inflammatory reactions.[3,9,55–57]

Parsons and colleagues[58] proposed the use of polymer-carbon fiber implants to provide a durable scaffold for the rapid ingrowth of collagen tissue after Achilles tendon rupture, theoretically allowing earlier rehabilitation and expedited return to function. Fifty-two chronic or acute Achilles tendon ruptures were repaired by weaving an absorbable polymer-carbon fiber ribbon between the proximal and distal tendon segments with 6 to 8 passes to bridge the defect. Augmentation with a turndown flap was left to the surgeon's discretion. They reported good or excellent outcomes in 86% of their cohort at an average of 2.1-years follow-up. The overall complication rate was 17.3%, including 2 reruptures, 2 deep infections, and 3 superficial infections. The use of carbon fiber in the repair of chronic and neglected Achilles tendon ruptures has been described in other cohorts with acceptable subject outcomes.[59] Despite satisfactory outcomes, histologic examinations in animal studies have demonstrated carbon fiber fragmentation, inflammatory response, and poor collagen deposition following implantation.[55]

Ozaki and colleagues[60] described the use of Marlex mesh to reconstruct neglected Achilles tendon ruptures in 6 subjects with defects ranging from 5 to 12 cm. All subjects demonstrated satisfactory outcomes with return to preinjury athletics. There were minimal signs of foreign-body reaction and adhesion to adjacent tissue. Satisfactory results have been demonstrated in another small case report using Ozaki and colleagues[60] technique.[61]

Jennings and Sefton[62] used polyester tape in 16 subjects with chronic ruptures. The polyester tape was passed through a 3.5 mm drill hole in the calcaneus and woven to the proximal tendon segment with a Bunnell-type stitch. Complications were reported in 5 subjects (31.3%), including 3 superficial wound infections, sural nerve injury, and revision surgery to remove the polyester tape. The proposed benefit of this technique is that it allows early weightbearing without the need for postoperative splint immobilization.[62,63]

The use of synthetic materials, including carbon fiber and Marlex mesh, has only been vetted in these small case series and can elicit an inflammatory response.[57–61] The authors do not think that the use of mesh replacements has been adequately studied and do not recommend this technique.

Allograft Dermal Patches

Acellular dermal human matrix can be used as a patch. The most commonly described technique is an onlay or circumferential Achilles wrap (burrito). This technique was used to augment end-to-end repair in 9 subjects with neglected Achilles tendon ruptures with good functional outcomes.[64] Cadaveric biomechanical studies have demonstrated an increase in the ultimate load to failure after direct end-to-end repair with acellular dermal human matrix augmentation.[65] The ultimate failure load in the control group (end-to-end repair alone) was 217 N plus or minus 31 compared with 455 N plus or minus 76.5 in the augmentation group (end-to-end repair with acellular dermal human matrix). The potential benefit of augmentation affords implementation of a more aggressive rehabilitation protocol and earlier return to activity without the concern for failure.[65]

The authors use dermal patches to augment a direct end-to end-repair in which the goal is early mobilization. The other indication is in a chronic rerupture in which the goal is to reestablish the paratenon that has been compromised due to infection or suture irritation. There are similar xenograft options commercially available. These grafts have acellular collagen matrix derived from sources such as equine pericardium[66] or porcine urinary bladder matrix.[67]

TENDON TRANSFERS

An ideal tendon transfer provides additional dynamic strength, reinforces the repair with physical substance, and provides increased vascularity to the repair.[68] The transferred tendon should function in phase with the Achilles during the gait cycle, minimizing the degree of neuromuscular retraining often required during the rehabilitation period. The tendon should be readily accessible and not lead to significant functional deficits after its harvest. Several tendon transfers have been used for neglected Achilles tendon ruptures, including the peroneus brevis, flexor digitorum longus (FDL), and the FHL. Each of these options has its own pertinent anatomy, advantages, and disadvantages that should be considered when deciding which tendon to transfer.

Gilcreest[69] first described using the plantaris tendon in 1933, leaving the calcaneal insertion intact. In 1966, Lynn[70] described a technique of detaching the plantaris tendon at its insertion and using its fibers to reinforce the Achilles tendon repair. Although effectively reinforcing the Achilles tendon repair, a plantaris tendon transfer does not provide improved plantarflexion strength. Therefore, the authors view plantaris tendon transfer more as an augmentation strategy rather than a dynamic tendon transfer and we do not recommend using the plantaris for chronic Achilles repairs.

The peroneus brevis tendon is a natural evertor of the foot that functions in phase with the Achilles tendon during the gait cycle. In 1974, Teuffer[71] described a technique of harvesting the peroneus brevis tendon, passing it through a bone tunnel in the calcaneus from lateral to medial and then suturing the tendon back to the proximal Achilles tendon. In 1987, Turco and Spinella[72] modified the Teuffer technique by passing the harvested peroneus brevis tendon through the distal Achilles stump rather than the calcaneus. They treated 24 neglected ruptures with this technique and reported subjective excellent outcomes. However, there are potential disadvantages associated with the peroneus brevis tendon transfer. Although the tendon transfer may be performed through the same skin incision, harvest of the peroneus brevis requires entering a separate muscle compartment. There is loss of eversion strength with a peroneus brevis tendon transfer. Furthermore, by placing the transferred tendon from lateral to medial through either the calcaneus or Achilles, the vector of pull does not match the native plantarflexion of the Achilles tendon. Proponents of the peroneus brevis tendon transfer argue that the peroneus longus tendon is more than twice as powerful as its counterpart, perhaps making the loss of eversion strength clinically insignificant.[73] In a cohort of 8 subjects treated for neglected Achilles tendon ruptures, there were no reported subjective complaints after peroneus brevis tendon transfer, despite a 14.9% loss of eversion strength.

FDL tendon transfer for neglected Achilles tendon ruptures was described by Mann and colleagues[74] in 1991. The FDL tendon was harvested through a separate midfoot incision. The distal FDL stump was sutured to the FHL tendon. The harvested FDL tendon was passed through the calcaneus from medial to lateral and then sewn back to itself and to the proximal Achilles tendon. A fascial turndown was also used to augment the Achilles repair. Six out of the 7 subjects demonstrated good or excellent results. The FDL functions in phase with the Achilles tendon during the gait cycle and it is also a natural plantar flexor. There is concern about weakened toe flexion and the development of lesser toe deformities with the harvest, but this has not been reported in the literature. Perhaps of more concern is potential injury to the adjacent neurovascular bundle because the FDL tendon transfer requires crossing the neurovascular bundle.

The most popular choice for tendon transfer in the setting of chronic Achilles tendon rupture repair is the FHL tendon. Hansen first described this technique, harvesting the FHL tendon through a single posterior skin incision.[75] Hansen described several potential advantages of using the FHL tendon. The FHL tendon lies within close proximity to the Achilles tendon, is a natural plantar flexor of the ankle, and functions in phase with the Achilles tendon. An additional advantage of this tendon for transfer is the closer proximity of the muscle belly to the repair site, which theoretically provides improved vascularity for healing. Wapner and colleagues[76] reported on a cohort of 7 chronic Achilles tendon ruptures treated with repair and FHL tendon transfer. They harvested the FHL through a separate midfoot incision, anchored the tendon through the calcaneus, and then wove the harvested tendon through the repaired Achilles tendon. Six of the subjects had good or excellent outcomes. They reported no functional deficits related to the FHL tendon harvest. The average plantarflexion strength was decreased by 29.5% compared with the uninjured side. Elias and colleagues[23] reported on 15 consecutive subjects treated for missed complete Achilles tendon ruptures with a 5-cm or larger tendon gap. They performed a V-Y advancement and an FHL tendon transfer through a single incision. The FHL tendon was anchored to the calcaneus through a bone tunnel directly anterior to the native Achilles tendon insertion. There was an average decrease in plantarflexion strength of 22.3%. All subjects were reportedly satisfied with their outcomes.

There is concern about the potential to develop hallux claw deformity, decreased great toe push-off strength, and transfer metatarsalgia following FHL tendon harvest. With a 2-incision harvest technique, there is also increased risk of medial or lateral plantar nerve injury. Using the single-incision technique, Den Hartog[77] published the outcomes of 26 subjects treated for chronic Achilles tendinosis. The FHL tendon was inserted into the calcaneus directly anterior to the native Achilles insertion site using a suture anchor. Twenty-three subjects demonstrated good or excellent results, with no reported functional deficits or deformities. Richardson and colleagues[78] reviewed 48 subjects who underwent single-incision FHL transfer for either chronic Achilles ruptures or Achilles tendinosis. They noted decreased plantar phalangeal pressures and FHL weakness. However, there was no difference in first and second metatarsal head plantar pressures. Their subjects had high functional outcome scores. Similarly, Coull and colleagues[79] found no significant changes in forefoot plantar pressures and good outcome scores with FHL tendon transfer. In 2008, Hahn and colleagues[80] reported on 13 subjects who underwent an FHL tendon transfer for chronic Achilles tendinopathy. They used a single-incision technique and wove the FHL tendon through the repaired Achilles tendon. All subjects reported a significant improvement in pain. There was an average decrease in plantarflexion strength of approximately 35%. All subjects underwent a follow-up MRI, with complete integration of the FHL tendon seen in 6 subjects. Ten subjects showed fatty atrophy of the triceps surae. No subjects showed signs of FHL degeneration and 8 subjects showed greater than 15% hypertrophy of the FHL tendon.

The FHL tendon transfer has proven to be a safe and effective adjunct for chronic Achilles tendon rupture repairs and the authors use this technique with great confidence when challenged by a chronically torn Achilles tendon.

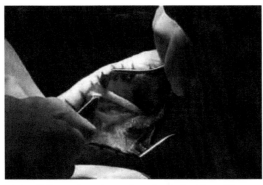

Fig. 6. Harvesting of the FHL tendon through a single incision. The great toe is maximally plantarflexed before transecting the tendon as far distally as can be visualized. (*From* Cottom JM, Hyer CF, Berlet GC, et al. Flexor hallucis tendon transfer with an interference screw for chronic Achilles tendinosis. Foot Ankle Spec 2008;1(5):283; with permission.)

AUTHORS' PREFERRED TECHNIQUE

The treatment goals for a chronic Achilles tendon tear are to close the gap of the tendon tear and re-establish a functional plantar flexion muscle unit.

The authors advocate direct end-to-end repair when the postdebridement gap is less than 2 cm and the repair can be achieved with a plantar flexion less than 30°. In some cases, we will augment this repair with an acellular dermis patch to improve strength.

When the ends cannot be repaired directly, we advocate a gastrocsoleus flap turn-down for the closure of the defect but will add an FHL tendon transfer to re-establish the plantar flexion power. When reapproximating the ends of the tendon requires plan-tarflexion of more than 20°, we will use a gastrocsoleus recession to help deliver the proximal end for an end-to-end repair. We no longer use the V-Y lengthening.

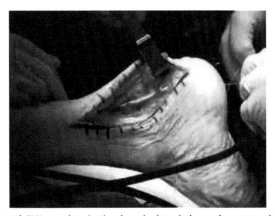

Fig. 7. The harvested FHL tendon is sized and placed through a tunnel in the calcaneus. With the ankle in about 10° of equinus, the tendon is secured in place with an interference screw. Note that the calcaneal insertion of the Achilles tendon has been removed, helping to demonstrate tunnel placement midline, anterior to native Achilles tendon insertion. (*From* Cottom JM, Hyer CF, Berlet GC, et al. Flexor hallucis tendon transfer with an interference screw for chronic Achilles tendinosis. Foot Ankle Spec 2008;1(5):286; with permission.)

We do not advocate allograft Achilles grafts, synthetic meshes or other autogenous sources external to the ankle for closure of the chronic defect.

We strongly advocate for an FHL tendon transfer harvested through a single posterior incision and anchored to the calcaneus with an interference screw as seen in **Figs. 6** and **7**. We do not believe that the extra length achieved with midfoot harvest is worth the added risk, scar, or extra operative time. We recommend that the FHL tendon transfer be kept separate from the chronically diseased Achilles tendon and do not advocate sewing these together. We do not believe that it is possible to achieve isometry between 2 unique contractile muscles (gastrocnemius-soleus and FHL), and instead allow each to achieve its own resting tone. We do not believe that suturing the FHL tendon to the Achilles brings new blood supply to a chronically diseased Achilles tendon.

The authors are optimistic that a patient with chronically torn Achilles tendon can be restored to good function and we define our preoperative expectations as the ability to wear regular shoe wear and regain the ability to do a single-heel rise.

REFERENCES

1. Myerson MS. Achilles tendon ruptures. Instr Course Lect 1999;48:219–30.
2. Ballas MT, Tytko J, Mannarino F. Commonly missed orthopedic problems. Am Fam Physician 1998;57(2):267–74.
3. Maffulli N, Ajis A. Management of chronic ruptures of the Achilles tendon. J Bone Joint Surg Am 2008;90(6):1348–60.
4. Leslie HD, Edwards WH. Neglected ruptures of the Achilles tendon. Foot Ankle Clin 2005;10(2):357–70.
5. Thompson TC. A test for rupture of the tendo achillis. Acta Orthop Scand 1962; 32:461–5.
6. Cuttica DJ, Hyer CF, Berlet GC. Intraoperative value of the thompson test. J Foot Ankle Surg 2015;54(1):99–101.
7. Matles AL. Rupture of the tendo achilles: another diagnostic sign. Bull Hosp Joint Dis 1975;36(1):48–51.
8. O'Brien T. The needle test for complete rupture of the Achilles tendon. J Bone Joint Surg Am 1984;66(7):1099–101.
9. Padanilam TG. Chronic Achilles tendon ruptures. Foot Ankle Clin 2009;14(4): 711–28.
10. Barnes MJ, Hardy AE. Delayed reconstruction of the calcaneal tendon. J Bone Joint Surg Br 1986;68(1):121–4.
11. Christensen I. Rupture of the Achilles tendon; analysis of 57 cases. Acta Chir Scand 1953;106(1):50–60.
12. Bruggeman NB, Turner NS, Dahm DL, et al. Wound complications after open Achilles tendon repair: an analysis of risk factors. Clin Orthop Relat Res 2004;(427):63–6.
13. Bullock MJ, DeCarbo WT, Hofbauer MH, et al. Repair of Chronic Achilles Ruptures Has a High Incidence of Venous Thromboembolism. Foot Ankle Spec 2016. [Epub ahead of print].
14. Uquillas CA, Guss MS, Ryan DJ, et al. Everything Achilles: knowledge update and current concepts in management: AAOS exhibit selection. J Bone Joint Surg Am 2015;97(14):1187–95.
15. Den Hartog BD. Surgical strategies: delayed diagnosis or neglected achilles' tendon ruptures. Foot Ankle Int 2008;29(4):456–63.
16. Kuwada GT. Classification of tendo Achillis rupture with consideration of surgical repair techniques. J Foot Surg 1990;29(4):361–5.

17. Porter DA, Mannarino FP, Snead D, et al. Primary repair without augmentation for early neglected Achilles tendon ruptures in the recreational athlete. Foot Ankle Int 1997;18(9):557–64.
18. Yasuda T, Shima H, Mori K, et al. Direct Repair of Chronic Achilles Tendon Ruptures Using Scar Tissue Located Between the Tendon Stumps. J Bone Joint Surg Am 2016;98(14):1168–75.
19. Bosworth DM. Repair of defects in the tendo achillis. J Bone Joint Surg Am 1956;38A(1):111–4.
20. Abraham E, Pankovich AM. Neglected rupture of the Achilles tendon. Treatment by V-Y tendinous flap. J Bone Joint Surg Am 1975;57(2):253–5.
21. Leitner A, Voigt C, Rahmanzadeh R. Treatment of extensive aseptic defects in old Achilles tendon ruptures: methods and case reports. Foot Ankle 1992;13(4):176–80.
22. Parker RG, Repinecz M. Neglected rupture of the achilles tendon. Treatment by modified Strayer gastrocnemius recession. J Am Podiatry Assoc 1979;69(9):548–55.
23. Elias I, Besser M, Nazarian LN, et al. Reconstruction for missed or neglected Achilles tendon rupture with V-Y lengthening and flexor hallucis longus tendon transfer through one incision. Foot Ankle Int 2007;28(12):1238–48.
24. Kissel CG, Blacklidge DK, Crowley DL. Repair of neglected Achilles tendon ruptures–procedure and functional results. J Foot Ankle Surg 1994;33(1):46–52.
25. Us AK, Bilgin SS, Aydin T, et al. Repair of neglected Achilles tendon ruptures: procedures and functional results. Arch Orthop Trauma Surg 1997;116(6–7):408–11.
26. Guclu B, Basat HC, Yildirim T, et al. Long-term Results of Chronic Achilles Tendon Ruptures Repaired With V-Y Tendon Plasty and Fascia Turndown. Foot Ankle Int 2016;37(7):737–42.
27. Strayer LM Jr. Recession of the gastrocnemius; an operation to relieve spastic contracture of the calf muscles. J Bone Joint Surg Am 1950;32A(3):671–6.
28. Strayer LM Jr. Gastrocnemius recession; five-year report of cases. J Bone Joint Surg Am 1958;40A(5):1019–30.
29. Arner O, Lindholm A. Subcutaneous rupture of the Achilles tendon; a study of 92 cases. Acta Chir Scand Suppl 1959;116(Supp 239):1–51.
30. Rush JH. Operative repair of neglected rupture of the tendo Achillis. Aust N Z J Surg 1980;50(4):420–2.
31. Ahmad J, Jones K, Raikin SM. Treatment of Chronic Achilles Tendon Ruptures With Large Defects. Foot Ankle Spec 2016;9(5):400–8.
32. Mao H, Shi Z, Xu D, et al. Neglected Achilles Tendon Rupture Treated with Flexor Hallucis Longus transfer with two turndown gastrocnemius fascia flap and reinforced with plantaris tendon. Acta Orthop Belg 2015;81(3):553–60.
33. Silfverskiold N. Uber die subkutane totale Achilles Sehnenruptur und deren Behandlung. Acta Chir Scand Suppl 1941;84:393–413.
34. Lindholm A. A new method of operation in subcutaneous rupture of the Achilles tendon. Acta Chir Scand 1959;117:261–70.
35. Takao M, Ochi M, Naito K, et al. Repair of neglected Achilles tendon rupture using gastrocnemius fascial flaps. Arch Orthop Trauma Surg 2003;123(9):471–4.
36. Lee YS, Lin CC, Chen CN, et al. Reconstruction for neglected Achilles tendon rupture: the modified Bosworth technique. Orthopedics 2005;28(7):647–50.
37. Gerdes MH, Brown TD, Bell AL, et al. A flap augmentation technique for Achilles tendon repair. Postoperative strength and functional outcome. Clin Orthop Relat Res 1992;(280):241–6.

38. Pajala A, Kangas J, Siira P, et al. Augmented compared with nonaugmented surgical repair of a fresh total Achilles tendon rupture. A prospective randomized study. J Bone Joint Surg Am 2009;91(5):1092–100.

39. Heikkinen J, Lantto I, Flinkkila T, et al. Augmented Compared with Nonaugmented Surgical Repair After Total Achilles Rupture: Results of a Prospective Randomized Trial with Thirteen or More Years of Follow-up. J Bone Joint Surg Am 2016; 98(2):85–92.

40. Cienfuegos A, Holgado MI, Diaz del Rio JM, et al. Chronic Achilles rupture reconstructed with Achilles tendon allograft: a case report. J Foot Ankle Surg 2013; 52(1):95–8.

41. Hanna T, Dripchak P, Childress T. Chronic achilles rupture repair by allograft with bone block fixation. technique tip. Foot Ankle Int 2014;35(2):168–74.

42. Hollawell S, Baione W. Chronic Achilles Tendon Rupture Reconstructed With Achilles Tendon Allograft and Xenograft Combination. J Foot Ankle Surg 2015; 54(6):1146–50.

43. Lepow GM, Green JB. Reconstruction of a neglected achilles tendon rupture with an achilles tendon allograft: A case report. J Foot Ankle Surg 2006;45(5):351–5.

44. Nellas ZJ, Loder BG, Wertheimer SJ. Reconstruction of an Achilles tendon defect utilizing an Achilles tendon allograft. J Foot Ankle Surg 1996;35(2):144–8 [discussion: 190].

45. Ofili KP, Pollard JD, Schuberth JM. The Neglected Achilles Tendon Rupture Repaired With Allograft: A Review of 14 Cases. J Foot Ankle Surg 2016;55(6): 1245–8.

46. Lewis JS Jr, Adams SB Jr, Nunley JA 2nd, et al. Allografts in foot and ankle surgery: a critical analysis review. JBJS Rev 2013;1(1) [pii:01874474-201311000-00002].

47. Tobin WJ. Repair of the neglected ruptured and severed Achilles tendon. Am Surg 1953;19(6):514–22.

48. Zadek I. Repair of old rupture of the tendo achillis by means of fascia lata: report of a case. J Bone Joint Surg Am 1940;22(4):1070–1.

49. Bugg EI Jr, Boyd BM. Repair of neglected rupture or laceration of the Achilles tendon. Clin Orthop Relat Res 1968;56:73–5.

50. Duhamel P, Mathieu L, Brachet M, et al. Reconstruction of the Achilles tendon with a composite anterolateral thigh free flap with vascularized fascia lata: a case report. J Bone Joint Surg Am 2010;92(15):2598–603.

51. Lee JW, Yu JC, Shieh SJ, et al. Reconstruction of the Achilles tendon and overlying soft tissue using antero-lateral thigh free flap. Br J Plast Surg 2000;53(7):574–7.

52. Maffulli N, Leadbetter WB. Free gracilis tendon graft in neglected tears of the achilles tendon. Clin J Sport Med 2005;15(2):56–61.

53. Maffulli N, Spiezia F, Testa V, et al. Free gracilis tendon graft for reconstruction of chronic tears of the Achilles tendon. J Bone Joint Surg Am 2012;94(10):906–10.

54. Dumbre Patil SS, Dumbre Patil VS, Basa VR, et al. Semitendinosus tendon autograft for reconstruction of large defects in chronic Achilles tendon ruptures. Foot Ankle Int 2014;35(7):699–705.

55. Amis AA, Campbell JR, Kempson SA, et al. Comparison of the structure of neotendons induced by implantation of carbon or polyester fibres. J Bone Joint Surg Br 1984;66(1):131–9.

56. Amis AA, Kempson SA, Campbell JR, et al. Anterior cruciate ligament replacement. Biocompatibility and biomechanics of polyester and carbon fibre in rabbits. J Bone Joint Surg Br 1988;70(4):628–34.

57. Basiglini L, Iorio R, Vadala A, et al. Achilles tendon surgical revision with synthetic augmentation. Knee Surg Sports Traumatol Arthrosc 2010;18(5):644–7.

58. Parsons JR, Weiss AB, Schenk RS, et al. Long-term follow-up of achilles tendon repair with an absorbable polymer carbon fiber composite. Foot Ankle 1989;9(4): 179–84.
59. Howard CB, Winston I, Bell W, et al. Late repair of the calcaneal tendon with carbon fibre. J Bone Joint Surg Br 1984;66(2):206–8.
60. Ozaki J, Fujiki J, Sugimoto K, et al. Reconstruction of neglected Achilles tendon rupture with Marlex mesh. Clin Orthop Relat Res 1989;(238):204–8.
61. Choksey A, Soonawalla D, Murray J. Repair of neglected Achilles tendon ruptures with Marlex mesh. Injury 1996;27(3):215–7.
62. Jennings AG, Sefton GK. Chronic rupture of tendo Achillis. Long-term results of operative management using polyester tape. J Bone Joint Surg Br 2002;84(3): 361–3.
63. Jennings AG, Sefton GK, Newman RJ. Repair of acute rupture of the Achilles tendon: a new technique using polyester tape without external splintage. Ann R Coll Surg Engl 2004;86(6):445–8.
64. Lee DK. Achilles tendon repair with acellular tissue graft augmentation in neglected ruptures. J Foot Ankle Surg 2007;46(6):451–5.
65. Barber FA, McGarry JE, Herbert MA, et al. A biomechanical study of Achilles tendon repair augmentation using GraftJacket matrix. Foot Ankle Int 2008; 29(3):329–33.
66. Grove JR, Hardy MA. Autograft, allograft and xenograft options in the treatment of neglected achilles tendon ruptures: a historical review with illustration of surgical repair. Foot Ankle J 2008;1(5).
67. Geiger SE, Deigni OA, Watson JT, et al. Management of open distal lower extremity wounds with exposed tendons using porcine urinary bladder matrix. Wounds 2016;28(9):306–16.
68. Lin JL. Tendon transfers for Achilles reconstruction. Foot Ankle Clin 2009;14(4): 729–44.
69. Gilcreest E. Ruptures and tears of muscles and tendons of the lower extremity: Report of fifteen cases. J Am Med Assoc 1933;100(3):153–60.
70. Lynn TA. Repair of the torn achilles tendon, using the plantaris tendon as a reinforcing membrane. J Bone Joint Surg Am 1966;48(2):268–72.
71. Perez Teuffer A. Traumatic rupture of the Achilles Tendon. Reconstruction by transplant and graft using the lateral peroneus brevis. Orthop Clin North Am 1974;5(1):89–93.
72. Turco VJ, Spinella AJ. Achilles tendon ruptures—peroneus brevis transfer. Foot Ankle 1987;7(4):253–9.
73. Gallant GG, Massie C, Turco VJ. Assessment of eversion and plantar flexion strength after repair of Achilles tendon rupture using peroneus brevis tendon transfer. Am J Orthop (Belle Mead NJ) 1995;24(3):257–61.
74. Mann RA, Holmes GB Jr, Seale KS, et al. Chronic rupture of the Achilles tendon: a new technique of repair. J Bone Joint Surg Am 1991;73(2):214–9.
75. Hansen S. Trauma to the heel cord. In: Jahss MH, editor. Disorders of the foot and ankle, vol. 3. Philadelphia: WB Saunders; 1991. p. 2355–60.
76. Wapner KL, Pavlock GS, Hecht PJ, et al. Repair of chronic Achilles tendon rupture with flexor hallucis longus tendon transfer. Foot Ankle 1993;14(8):443–9.
77. Den Hartog BD. Flexor hallucis longus transfer for chronic Achilles tendonosis. Foot Ankle Int 2003;24(3):233–7.
78. Richardson DR, Willers J, Cohen BE, et al. Evaluation of the hallux morbidity of single-incision flexor hallucis longus tendon transfer. Foot Ankle Int 2009;30(7): 627–30.

79. Coull R, Flavin R, Stephens MM. Flexor hallucis longus tendon transfer: evaluation of postoperative morbidity. Foot Ankle Int 2003;24(12):931–4.

80. Hahn F, Meyer P, Maiwald C, et al. Treatment of chronic achilles tendinopathy and ruptures with flexor hallucis tendon transfer: clinical outcome and MRI findings. Foot Ankle Int 2008;29(8):794–802.

Treatment of Neglected Achilles Tendon Ruptures with Interpositional Allograft

 CrossMark

Christopher E. Gross, MD[a],*, James A. Nunley, MD[b]

KEYWORDS

- Chronic Achilles tear • Achilles allograft • Achilles reconstruction

KEY POINTS

- At 4 weeks, the Achilles is thought to be chronically torn because the tendon may have a fibrovascular scar that may trick surgeons because patients will no longer have a palpable defect at the rupture site.
- Any persistently symptomatic patient with an Achilles tendon rupture more than 6 weeks old with appropriate treatment who is seen in the office is a surgical candidate.
- No evidence-based algorithm exists to help with repairing neglected ruptures. There are a variety of treatment options that all have valid uses but have not been proven to be superior to one another.
- In larger defects greater than 6 cm, the authors prefer to reconstruct the Achilles tendon with an allograft with or without the use of synthetic graft augmentation.

INTRODUCTION

The Achilles tendon is the most commonly ruptured tendon in the body[1]; it accounts for 20% of all large tendon injuries.[2] Although most astute clinicians can diagnose Achilles tendon ruptures by physical examination alone,[3] more than 20% are not accurately diagnosed in a timely fashion.[4]

The definition of a "chronic" Achilles tendon rupture in foot and ankle literature varies widely: from 4 to 10 weeks after injury.[5] At the authors' institutions, they consider 4 weeks to be the cutoff, because ruptures as early as 6 weeks may have a fibrovascular scar that must be removed before repair.[5] This scar may trick surgeons into thinking that the Achilles has actually healed because patients will no longer have a palpable defect at the rupture site; at the same time, most will have

The authors have nothing to disclose.
[a] Department of Orthopaedics, Medical University of South Carolina, 96 Jonathan Lucas Drive, CSB 708, MSC 622, Charleston, SC 29425, USA; [b] Department of Orthopaedic Surgery, Duke University Medical Center, 4709 Creekstone Drive, Durham, NC 27703, USA
* Corresponding author.
E-mail address: cgross144@gmail.com

gained some plantarflexion strength because of recruitment of other ankle plantarflexors. Biomechanically, the scar actually lengthens the gastrocnemius-soleus tendon unit—relaxing the muscle-tendon complex and rendering the Achilles weak. This scar is incapable of acting as a tension band when the ankle is dorsiflexed and is also unable to contract contractile forces when the ankle is plantarflexed.

Neglected or chronic Achilles tendon ruptures can be significantly disabling to patients if the muscle-tendon unit is stretched beyond its normal passive limit. Patients may have significant balance and gait problems, with particular difficulty when ascending stairs or walking up inclines. Similarly, large areas of Achilles tendinopathy can lead to deterioration in functional structure of the muscle tendon unit.

Clinical Findings

Diagnosing an Achilles tendon rupture is largely a clinical diagnosis that can be made without the use of advanced imaging. A detailed history and physical examination can lead to the correct diagnosis in most patients. Patients may recall a remote history of a popping sensation in the posterior aspect of their distal leg after pushing off from a dorsiflexed position. Intense pain may eventually give way to a dull ache after a few hours; the patient is left with weak plantarflexion and a gait disturbance with difficulty bearing weight.

After 2 weeks, the frayed tendon edges become thickened with scar tissue and can be fibrosed to the overlying paratenon and fascia. The proximal tendon stump is often adherent to the flexor hallucis muscle belly (FHL), which causes a further reduction in plantarflexion strength.[6]

On inspection, the gastrocnemius-soleus muscles are often atrophied. The toe flexors are often recruited to make up for plantarflexion strength. A contracted flexor digitorum longus may cause a higher medial arch and clawing of the lesser toes.

The American Academy of Orthopaedic Surgeons Clinical Practice Guidelines[7] recommend that the diagnosis of Achilles tendon rupture can be made with 2 or more of the following physical examination findings: positive Thompson test, decreased plantarflexion strength, palpable tendon defect, and increased passive ankle dorsiflexion. When the patient is supine, one can examine the strength of plantar flexion and may feel a palpable gap in the tendon. When the Achilles is disrupted, one can still weakly plantarflex with the secondary plantarflexors. Chronically, the clinician may be confused by the pseudotendon that bridges the tendon stumps and gives the false impression of a tendon in continuity. Once prone, resting tension is measured and the Thompson test is carried out. The patient is then turned prone with the knees at a 90° flexion angle. First, the resting tension (Matles test) of the affected leg is observed (see **Fig. 2**). Both the Matles test and the Thompson test are highly sensitive.[8]

Imaging studies have a limited role in diagnosing a chronic rupture and should only be routinely used if the clinical diagnosis is uncertain. If one wishes to plan for an allograft reconstruction, one must pay attention to T2-weighted images, which may show fatty atrophy of the gastrocnemius soleus. More than 30% of fibrofatty atrophy in the muscle is a contraindication to allograft replacement.

Treatment Goals

A chronic Achilles tendon rupture is a functional burden. Postinjury changes of morphology and kinematics were noted in the nonathletic population. At 11 years after rupture, Horstmann and colleagues[9] noted smaller values of the injured side's calf circumference, ankle range of motion, and heel height during heel-raise tests as compared with the uninjured leg. This report underscores the observation that after repair of the ruptured Achilles tendon, muscle atrophy is a long-term consideration.[10] The treatment goal of repairing the chronic rupture is to restore the muscle-tendon complex, such that the Achilles can again act as a powerful plantarflexor such that patients may resume their desired levels of activity.

Nonoperative Treatment

Any persistently symptomatic patient with an Achilles tendon rupture more than 6 weeks old with appropriate treatment (immobilization in plantarflexion) who is seen in the office is a surgical candidate.[11]

Operative Management

Although some surgeons have conceptualized managing chronic Achilles tendon injuries,[12,13] no evidence-based algorithm exists to help with repairing neglected ruptures. There are a variety of treatment options that all have valid uses, but they have not been proven to be superior to one another. In larger defects greater than 6 cm, the authors prefer to reconstruct the Achilles tendon with an allograft with or without the use of synthetic graft augmentation.

AUTHORS' PREFERRED TREATMENT

- Indications:
  - Achilles tendons that have not healed and cause pain and a decrease in function
  - Those who would be less functional and active with a flexor hallucis longus transfer
- Contraindications:
  - Those with a poor posterior soft-tissue envelope
  - Poorly controlled diabetics with peripheral neuropathy
  - Medical comorbidities that contraindicate all surgery
  - Fatty atrophy of the gastrocnemius-soleus complex on MRI

Surgical Technique

Anesthesia

- Most importantly, the femoral and sciatic divisions must be blocked. Therefore, several permutations achieve this goal.
- General (or spinal) + popliteal block; general (or spinal) + popliteal + muscle relaxation; femoral + sciatic block; popliteal + saphenous; femoral + popliteal

Positioning

- Before the patient is placed on the operative table, a well-padded thigh tourniquet is placed on the operative leg and inflated after exsanguination.
- The patient is placed prone onto a radiolucent operative table.
  - Padding is placed under the anterior superior iliac crest, the level of the chest, and at the knees.
- The operation is facilitated by having the involved extremity placed on multiple flat blankets to provide a solid operating surface while keeping the leg elevated above the opposite extremity to facilitate lateral radiographs.
  - The ankle should be at roughly 30° of plantarflexion.
- The contralateral ankle may be prepared for comparison of resting plantar flexion.

Approach

- An incision is made directly over the midline of the Achilles tendon starting 20 cm proximal to the insertion site and extending to the glabrous skin of the heel.
- The paratenon is gently separated from the scar of the ruptured tendon from proximal to distal. Retractors are placed.
- Once this is done, the scarred Achilles tendon can be freed up in total.
- At this point, the proximal end of the distal tendon is palpated and is transected at a point where it is thought to be normal tendon.
- Then proximally, the muscle is stretched distally to gain back some of the myostatic contracture. It helpful to use Allis clamps or to pull the tendon with a sponge wrapped around it.
- Then the proximal tendon is transected at a point where the tendon is felt to be normal.
- The tendon gap is measured between the conical proximal stump and the bulbous distal stump.
    - If the tendon ends are less than 3 cm apart, an end-to-end repair is undertaken as described in Elizabeth Harkin and colleagues' article, "Treatment of acute and chronic tibialis anterior tendon rupture and tendinopathy," in this issue
    - If the ends are greater than 6 cm apart, then an Achilles allograft reconstruction is performed.
- The allograft tendon (usually peroneus longus) is then thawed and rehydrated in room temperature saline solution.
- The proximal Achilles tendon is divided with a fish-mouth opening over a distance of about 6 cm (Pulvertaft weave).
    - This maneuver allows the allograft to fan out so it can be attached proximally.
- The peroneus longus proximal portion is sutured to the Achilles tendon with 0 Tycron sutures with multiple strands so the fish mouth is closed over the allograft to get strong fixation.
- Distally, a no. 15 blade is used to create a lateral-to-medial tunnel through the distal stump.
- The distal portion of the allograft tendon is then passed through the Achilles tendon and up the proximal musculotendinous junction.
- The foot is set in plantarflexion, and the tension is adjusted in what is felt to be equal to the contralateral leg.
- The end of the allograft tendon (that is now looped through the Achilles distally and brought back up to proximal portion) is then sutured with 0 Tycron suture to the distal stump.
- The distal end of the allograft is attached via a Pulvertaft weave technique when the tension is found to be satisfactory.
- The fanned-out portion of the peroneus longus is wrapped around the second strand to create a thicker tendon and is sutured with a 0 Vicryl suture (**Fig. 1**).
- To augment the repair, an acellular dermal matrix can be wrapped around the construct as a cylinder and is sutured with a 2-0 Vicryl tendon (**Fig. 2**).
- The wound is irrigated and the paratenon is closed with 2-0 Vicryl suture over a medium Hemovac.
- After using a no-touch technique of closing the skin with 4-0 Nylon vertical mattress sutures, a Bulky Jones splint is placed.

Postoperative protocol

The authors' postoperative protocol includes a bulky dressing splinted in plantar flexion for 2 weeks with subsequent suture removal. The patient is then placed in a

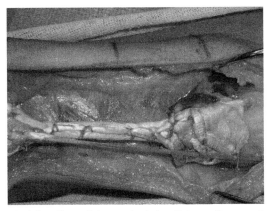

Fig. 1. The distal end of the allograft is attached via a Pulvertaft weave technique when the tension is found to be satisfactory. The fanned out portion of the peroneus longus is wrapped around the second strand to create a thicker tendon. This is sutured with a 0 Vicryl suture.

short-leg non-weight-bearing cast in slight plantarflexion for 4 more weeks. At 6 weeks postoperatively, the patient is placed into a CAM boot weight-bearing with CAM boot removal for plantarflexion exercises only. At 10 to 12 weeks, the patient transitions into a shoe with a 1-cm heel wedge, and physical therapy is then initiated for wound mobilization, scar adhesions, gentle range of motion, and free active range of motion. The patient may begin to use a recumbent bicycle, pool exercises, and a deweighted treadmill. At 12 to 14 weeks postoperatively, progressive strengthening and stretching are started. If the patient does well from a physical therapy standpoint, the patient is allowed to wear an athletic shoe and begin full-impact activities at 6 months. Ultimately, the patient should be able to perform a single-limb heel raise (**Fig. 3**).

Pearl

- The final tension of the operative ankle should be slightly more than the unaffected ankle to account for soft tissue relaxation.

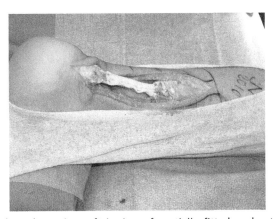

Fig. 2. Acellular dermal matrix graft is circumferentially fitted and sutured around the repaired tendon construct.

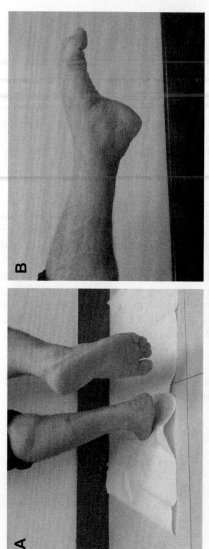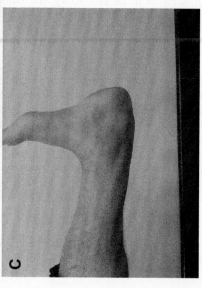

Fig. 3. A 35-year-old man 2 years after Achilles reconstruction demonstrating single-limb heel raise (A), plantarflexion (B), and dorsiflexion (C).

OUTCOMES

Allograft reconstruction in the foot and ankle is becoming popular for treating chronic ruptures and tendinopathy, specifically of the peroneals and anterior tibial tendon.[14] In many case reports[15–24] and a few case series,[25–27] allograft reconstruction has proven useful for treating chronic Achilles ruptures. Using an allograft is advantageous in that it does not have any risk of donor site morbidity, and the muscle-tendon unit tension can be adjusted with relative ease. Using this technique, one does not have to sacrifice a normally functioning muscle, like the FHL. It allows healing to occur outside the "watershed area" where vascular compromise is common (4–6 cm proximal to insertion of Achilles). In addition, using allograft tendon, the authors span the defect with naturally rotating tendon fibers, which may improve the overall function of plantarflexion, although this effect is unclear. With allograft, however, there is a chance for immunologic rejection and the spread of blood-borne diseases.

Case reports describe a variety of methods of using Achilles allograft, as follows:

- Interpositional Achilles allograft[20,21] (freeze-dried or fresh-frozen)
- Interpositional fascia lata allograft[23]
- Calcaneal bone block-Achilles tendon allograft[16,17,19]
- Sural fasciocutaneous flap and calcaneal bone block-tendon allograft[18]
- Flexor hallucis transfer and calcaneal bone block-tendon allograft[15]
- Interpositional Achilles allograft plus rectus muscle free flap[24]
- Adipofascial sural turnover flap and gracillis tendon allograft[22]

Interpositional Allografts

In a case report describing the use of an interpositional Achilles tendon allograft, Nellas and colleagues[21] used 2 strips of freeze-dried Achilles allograft to reconstruct a 4.5-cm tendon defect, following a debridement of an infected primary rupture repair. Although the patient had decreased strength at 2.5 years postsurgery, the patient had a good functional result. Hollawell and Baione[26] described a series of 4 patients who underwent treatment of chronic Achilles tendon ruptures with Achilles interpositional allograft and xenograft augmentation. After debriding the Achilles pseudotendon, the allograft was seated directly into the defect site and repaired intrasubstance with 2-0 nonabsorbable braided polyethylene suture (with the ankle in slight plantarflexion). Once the allograft was in place, a purified collagen matrix was used to augment the repair sites. All patients returned to work at a mean of 14.3 weeks with preinjury levels of activity. No complications, including rerupture, were reported.

Bone Block Allografts

In another technique article, Hanna and colleagues[17] used Achilles tendon allograft with a calcaneal bone block for patients with either chronic ruptures or tendinopathy. Once the diseased Achilles tendon was excised, the patient's native posterosuperior calcaneus was osteotomized in a distal-posterior to proximal-anterior direction. When the host and graft bone blocks were cut to size, the ankle was brought into plantarflexion and the bone block was fixated with 2- to 4.5-mm cannulated screws with washers. The graft was tensioned and repaired to the native tendon at the appropriate tension. In this series of 6 patients, all had satisfactory outcomes, although 4 out of 6 had subjective weakness. All patients were able to do a single heel raise and all had 5/5 strength. All patients had a normal range of motion.

Deese and colleagues[25] reported on a series of 8 patients, with an average age of 46 years, with either chronically ruptured or tendinopathic Achilles tendons who also underwent a calcaneal bone block reconstruction (fresh-frozen) in a technique similar to Hanna and colleagues.[17] The mean gap repaired was 7.9 cm. Three patients had complications: one patient fragmented the calcaneal tuberosity at 4 weeks; another had 3 cm of delayed wound healing; and another patient had radiographic evidence of retrocalcaneal heterotopic bone next to the allograft. Eight out of 9 patients had good functional status at last outcome with patients reporting no pain.

Ofili and colleagues[27] described the largest series of Achilles tendon ruptures treated either with an Achilles allograft alone (12 patients) or with a bone block and tendon allograft (2 patients). The mean interval from injury to surgery was 6.9 months with the mean intraoperative defect size after debridement of 7.0 cm. All 14 patients were able to perform a single heel raise at a mean of 27 weeks postoperatively. There were no complications except for a delayed union of a bone block, which eventually healed at 12 weeks. This group used MRI scans to try to determine gap length preoperatively. They noted that in each case, the MRI underestimated the true defect.

SUMMARY

The treatment of chronic or neglected Achilles tendon ruptures can be challenging. Fortunately, the foot and ankle surgeon has a wide array of surgical techniques in his armamentarium, with an interpositional Achilles allograft useful for the largest defects. Surgeons should try to improve existing techniques and create prospective, randomized trials to determine the best treatments for patients.

REFERENCES

1. Maffulli N. Rupture of the Achilles tendon. J Bone Joint Surg Am 1999;81(7): 1019–36.
2. Gillies H, Chalmers J. The management of fresh ruptures of the tendo achillis. J Bone Joint Surg Am 1970;52(2):337–43.
3. DiStefano VJ, Nixon JE. Achilles tendon rupture: pathogenesis, diagnosis, and treatment by a modified pullout wire technique. J Trauma 1972;12(8):671–7.
4. Maffulli N. Clinical tests in sports medicine: more on Achilles tendon. Br J Sports Med 1996;30(3):250.
5. Porter DA, Mannarino FP, Snead D, et al. Primary repair without augmentation for early neglected Achilles tendon ruptures in the recreational athlete. Foot Ankle Int 1997;18(9):557–64.
6. Maffulli N, Leadbetter WB. Free gracilis tendon graft in neglected tears of the achilles tendon. Clin J Sport Med 2005;15(2):56–61.
7. Chiodo CP, Glazebrook M, Bluman EM, et al. Diagnosis and treatment of acute Achilles tendon rupture. J Am Acad Orthop Surg 2010;18(8):503–10.
8. Maffulli N. The clinical diagnosis of subcutaneous tear of the Achilles tendon. A prospective study in 174 patients. Am J Sports Med 1998;26(2):266–70.
9. Horstmann T, Lukas C, Merk J, et al. Deficits 10-years after Achilles tendon repair. Int J Sports Med 2012;33(6):474–9.
10. Leppilahti J, Lahde S, Forsman K, et al. Relationship between calf muscle size and strength after achilles rupture repair. Foot Ankle Int 2000;21(4):330–5.
11. Maffulli N, Ajis A, Longo UG, et al. Chronic rupture of tendo Achillis. Foot Ankle Clin 2007;12(4):583–96, vi.
12. Kuwada GT. Classification of tendo Achillis rupture with consideration of surgical repair techniques. J Foot Surg 1990;29(4):361–5.
13. Myerson MS. Achilles tendon ruptures. Instr Course Lect 1999;48:219–30.

14. Mook WR, Parekh SG, Nunley JA. Allograft reconstruction of peroneal tendons: operative technique and clinical outcomes. Foot Ankle Int 2013;34(9):1212–20.
15. Catanzariti AR, Hentges M. Combined tendon and bone allograft transplantation for chronic Achilles tendon ruptures. Clin Podiatr Med Surg 2016;33(1):125–37.
16. Cienfuegos A, Holgado MI, Diaz del Rio JM, et al. Chronic Achilles rupture reconstructed with Achilles tendon allograft: a case report. J Foot Ankle Surg 2013; 52(1):95–8.
17. Hanna T, Dripchak P, Childress T. Chronic Achilles rupture repair by allograft with bone block fixation: technique tip. Foot Ankle Int 2014;35(2):168–74.
18. Hansen U, Moniz M, Zubak J, et al. Achilles tendon reconstruction after sural fasciocutaneous flap using Achilles tendon allograft with attached calcaneal bone block. J Foot Ankle Surg 2010;49(1):86.e5-10.
19. Haraguchi N, Bluman EM, Myerson MS. Reconstruction of chronic Achilles tendon disorders with Achilles tendon allograft. Tech Foot Ankle Surg 2005;4: 154–9.
20. Lepow GM, Green JB. Reconstruction of a neglected achilles tendon rupture with an Achilles tendon allograft: a case report. J Foot Ankle Surg 2006;45(5):351–5.
21. Nellas ZJ, Loder BG, Wertheimer SJ. Reconstruction of an Achilles tendon defect utilizing an Achilles tendon allograft. J Foot Ankle Surg 1996;35(2): 144–8 [discussion: 190].
22. Parodi PC, Moretti L, Saggin G, et al. Soft tissue and tendon reconstruction after achilles tendon rupture: adipofascial sural turnover flap associated withcryopreserved gracilis tendon allograft for complicated soft tissue and achilles tendon losses. A case report and literature review. Ann Ital Chir 2006;77(4):361–7.
23. Saxena V, Pradhan P, Yadav A, et al. Reconstruction of bilateral tendoachilles with fascia lata graft. Indian J Orthop 2013;47(6):634–8.
24. Yuen JC, Nicholas R. Reconstruction of a total Achilles tendon and soft-tissue defect using an Achilles allograft combined with a rectus muscle free flap. Plast Reconstr Surg 2001;107(7):1807–11.
25. Deese JM, Gratto-Cox G, Clements FD, et al. Achilles allograft reconstruction for chronic achilles tendinopathy. J Surg Orthop Adv 2015;24(1):75–8.
26. Hollawell S, Baione W. Chronic Achilles tendon rupture reconstructed with Achilles tendon allograft and xenograft combination. J Foot Ankle Surg 2015; 54(6):1146–50.
27. Ofili KP, Pollard JD, Schuberth JM. The neglected Achilles tendon rupture repaired with allograft: a retrospective review of 14 cases. J Foot Ankle Surg 2016. http://dx.doi.org/10.1053/j.jfas.2016.01.001.

Noninsertional Tendinopathy of the Achilles

Avreeta Singh, MD, Arash Calafi, MD, Chris Diefenbach, MD,
Chris Kreulen, MD, Eric Giza, MD*

KEYWORDS

- Achilles tendinopathy • Achilles tendinosis • Noninsertional tendinopathy
- Noninsertional Achilles tendinosis

KEY POINTS

- The clinical triad of pain, swelling, and decreased performance ability indicates the diagnosis of Achilles tendinopathy.
- The current understanding of the etiology likely involves a combination of overuse leading to repetitive microtrauma, poor vascularity of the tissue, mechanical imbalances of the extremity, genetic predisposition, and a variety of metabolic factors.
- Conservative measures are generally recommended as the initial treatment strategy with an attempt to address and correct some of the underlying etiologic factors, followed by activity modification, medications, and stretching/strengthening programs.
- Surgery is considered an acceptable option for patients who do not respond to conservative measures.

INTRODUCTION

Noninsertional Achilles tendinosis is a condition that causes a predictable triad of symptoms, including pain, swelling over the affected site, and decreased performance ability. Achilles tendinosis must first be differentiated based on anatomic location—it can be subdivided into insertional (arising at the tendo-Achilles junction) or noninsertional (located 2–6 cm proximal to this Achilles insertion).[1,2] It is also important to differentiate between tendonitis and tendinosis with regards to Achilles pathology. Tendonitis refers to primarily an inflammatory response within the tendon after mechanical overloading, typically in an acute setting. Tendinosis on the other hand is primarily a degenerative process referring to a chronic overuse phenomenon whereby repetitive strains cause repeated tears and degeneration. Thus, the tissue's inability to adequately heal perpetuates pain and functional limitations and the role of inflammation although controversial is thought to be limited.[3,4] This has important implications in treatment approaches, which are discussed.

The authors have nothing to disclose.
University of California, Davis, 4860 Y Street, Suite 1700, Sacramento, CA 95817, USA
* Corresponding author.
E-mail address: ericgiza@gmail.com

Foot Ankle Clin N Am 22 (2017) 745–760
http://dx.doi.org/10.1016/j.fcl.2017.07.006
1083-7515/17/© 2017 Elsevier Inc. All rights reserved.

foot.theclinics.com

EPIDEMIOLOGY

Achilles tendinosis is frequently seen in the athletic population and is associated with activities that require running and jumping. Achilles tendinopathy can also be found among patients who do not participate in sports.[5,6] High prevalence in runners has been reported in studies with prevalence ranging between 8% and 9%.[7–12] Similar to degenerative changes seen elsewhere in the musculoskeletal system, it is likely that many individuals have histologic findings of tendinosis, but are asymptomatic throughout their lifetime.

ETIOLOGY

The exact etiology of noninsertional Achilles tendinosis is unclear. Several explanations have been proposed, and it is likely a multifactorial process. In the future, the relative impact of the different contributing factors will need to be elucidated. Broadly, these factors can be categorized into the framework of intrinsic (ie, age, gender, body mass index, biomechanical abnormalities, foot malalignment, gastrocnemius-soleus dysfunction, ankle instability, and so forth) and extrinsic (ie, steroid use, fluoroquinolones, improper training, environmental factors, footwear, and so forth) factors.[13] Several pathophysiologic processes thought to be associated with tendinosis are discussed.

Mechanical Injury

Mechanical injury to the tendon is the inciting stimulus toward pathology. It may arise from physiologic overloading of the tendon or by accumulation of multiple physiologic loads without adequate healing. Healing in the setting of the Achilles tendon is likely mediated by tenocytes that detect alterations in the extracellular matrix. It has been suggested that failure to restore this extracellular matrix may result in release of cytokines that further modulate tenocyte activity and inhibit proper healing creating a degenerative spiral.[14]

Activities that require strong repetitive toe push-off forces, such as running and jumping, generate both tensile and torsional forces and predispose an individual to overuse and increased mechanical loads up to 9000 N.[15,16] Although an acute overload may result in an inflammation of the synovial sheath of the Achilles (as in tendinitis), repetitive physiologic loads without adequate healing predispose to degenerative changes within the tendon substance itself.[17,18]

Vascular Anatomy

Proponents of a vascular etiology for Achilles tendinosis suggest that pathology stems from the unique pattern of flow to the Achilles tendon. Although this topic has been investigated many times, there is no uniform consensus regarding either the Achilles' exact vascular topography or the uniformity of its flow.[19–23]

Chen and colleagues[24] performed an anatomic, histologic, and angiographic cadaveric study and concluded that the Achilles tendon is supplied by 2 arteries, the posterior tibial and peroneal arteries. They designated 3 vascular areas, with the midsection supplied by the peroneal artery and the proximal and distal sections supplied by the posterior tibial artery. They noted that the midsection of the Achilles tendon was markedly more hypovascular that the rest of the tendon in all specimens. From this they suggested the midsection of the Achilles was at highest risk for rupture as well as complications after surgery.

Astrom and Westlin[25] conducted a study looking at blood flow specifically in patients with chronic Achilles tendinopathy compared with normal controls. They used laser Doppler flowmetry at rest and during physical provocation by passive stretch and contraction of the gastroc-soleus complex. They noted values that were significantly lower at the distal insertion but otherwise evenly distributed throughout the tendon. More interestingly, and contrary to the widely held belief that pathologic tendons have poorer perfusion, they found that diseased tendons actually had overall increased blood flow throughout the tendon.[25] Based on these conflicting studies, it seems that further work into understanding importance of vascularity in the pathophysiology of the disease remains to be done.

Metabolic Factors

Metabolic factors, such as hypertension, hyperlipidemia, and obesity, have all been shown to predispose to Achilles tendinopathy and rupture.[26,27] It has been proposed that all these factors work through a common pathway of decreased tissue vascularity and subsequently diminished tissue healing potential.[28,29] Both hypertension and obesity have been shown to decrease levels of nitric oxide, one pathway used to establish vascular dilation and increase blood flow.[28]

Diabetes mellitus contributes to diminished vascularity, primarily at the microvascular level, which can compromise the normal metabolism and reparative ability of the Achilles tendon. Diabetes is also thought to increase advanced glycation end-products on tissues, changing tissue properties and resulting in increased stiffness.[30,31]

Other Factors

Multiple other factors, with poorly understood mechanisms, have been suggested as contributing to tendinopathy. These include increasing age[32] and certain drugs, such as quinolones, long-term glucocorticoids, statins, and aromatase inhibitors.[33] Moreover, certain mechanical factors, including hyperpronation of the foot,[15] decreased motion at the ankle and subtalar joints,[34] varus deformity of the forefoot,[15,35] and limb length discrepancies,[36] have been suggested as contributing to pathology.

BIOLOGY AND HISTOLOGY

Normal Achilles cellular composition is almost exclusively tenocytes and tenoblasts (90%–95%), with the remaining cellular contents comprising chondrocytes, vascular, synovial, and smooth muscle cells. The extracellular matrix component is composed of collagen (primarily type 1) and elastin fibers, ground substance, and organic components, such as calcium.[37] As degenerative changes occur to the tissue, however, the cellular and extracellular composition and the histologic appearance of the tissue change. Specimens of pathologic Achilles tendons have been found to have abnormalities of their collagen fibers (abnormal variations in diameter, disintegration, and longitudinal splitting), cystic mucoid changes (large mucoid patches and vacuoles between thin, fragile collagen fibers), tendolipomatosis (lipid cells interspersed within collagen fibers), and calcific deposits as well as vascular changes.[12] Much work is being done on the biochemical and genetic changes that occur as the tendon transitions from healthy to diseased. Alfredson and colleagues[38] found interesting gene expression differences between healthy and diseased tendons, specifically upregulation of matrix metalloproteinase 2, fibronectin subunit B, vascular endothelial growth factor, and mitogen-activated protein kinase p38 and down-regulation of matrix metalloproteinase 3 and decorin.

PATIENT EVALUATION/DIAGNOSIS

Typically, a patient presents with pain localized 2 cm to 6 cm proximal to the calcaneal insertion, particularly with exercise. The discomfort is increased at beginning and end of exercise sessions, with an intermediate period of minimized discomfort. On examination the hindfoot must be evaluated for malalignment, deformity, tendon asymmetry, thickening, Haglund deformity, and previous scarring. Fusiform swelling of the Achilles tendon 4 cm to 6 cm proximal to the calcaneal insertion can be found (**Fig. 1**). On palpation, tenderness, heat, thickening, nodularity, or crepitus may be found in the affected area. Painful range of motion can be found, which is characterized by movement of the nodule within the paratenon during plantar/dorsiflexion.[39–44]

Appropriate imaging plays a role in the diagnosis and treatment plan. Plain film lateral radiograph is useful because it may show an associated bony abnormality or intrasubstance calcification (**Fig. 2**). The use of MRI or ultrasound should be considered on a case-by-case basis to gain more information on the internal tendon morphology and is useful for preoperative planning: extent of degeneration and peritendinitis versus tendinosis. Sagittal and axial MRI images are helpful to determine the percentage of tendon involvement because augmentation may be necessary if greater than 50% of the tendon is removed (**Fig. 3**). The disease process results in disorganized tissue, which appears as intrasubstance intermediate signal intensity (**Tables 1** and **2**).

NONPHARMALOGIC TREATMENT OPTIONS

The goals of treatment in the early phase of the condition are to control inflammation. Conservative measures are generally recommended as the initial treatment strategy.

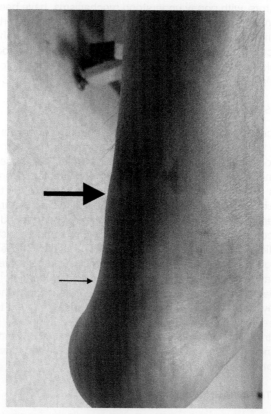

Fig. 1. Clinical photo demonstrating a fusiform swelling of an Achilles tendon 4 cm proximal to the calcaneus (*large arrow*) contrasted with the normal width of the Achilles (*small arrow*).

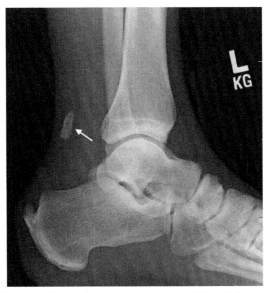

Fig. 2. Lateral radiograph of the ankle demonstrating an intrasubstance calcification in the center of an area of midsubstance tendinopathy (*arrow*).

An attempt to address and possibly correct some of the underlying etiologic factors should be made, followed by a multimodal approach, including activity modification, medications, and stretching/strengthening programs.[44–46] The inflammation usually present during the early phase of Achilles tendinopathy is best addressed with the use of cryotherapy and decreasing activity. Sometimes these simple changes are

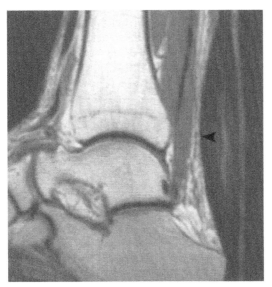

Fig. 3. Sagittal T1-weighted MRI demonstrating a thickened Achilles tendon with altered signal intensity within the central tendon *(arrowhead)*.

Table 1
Nonpharmacologic treatment options for noninsertional Achilles tendinopathy

Intervention	Evidence	Conclusion
Stretching	One level I study	No definitive conclusion possible
Cryotherapy	Level IV studies	No definitive conclusion possible
Eccentric training	Multiple level I studies	Strong evidence in support
ESWT	Multiple level I studies	Moderate evidence in support

sufficient to control the inflammation and painful symptoms associated with acute tendinopathy.[47–49]

Eccentric exercise is the cornerstone for conservative management of Achilles tendinopathy. Its method of action is still poorly understood but postulated as related to its ability to disrupt neovascularization by shear forces between the paratenon-fascial-tendon layers.[50,51] With the hypothesis that neovascular ingrowth is related to pain, researchers have also demonstrated a reduction in the neovascular make-up of the tendon after a 12-week course of eccentric exercises.[52] Night splinting has not been shown beneficial.[53–55]

PHARMACOLOGIC TREATMENT OPTIONS

Nonsteroidal anti-inflammatory drugs (NSAIDs) are commonly recommended pharmacologic treatment of tendinopathies; however, the scientific basis for NSAID use for these conditions is controversial. Some studies have indicated that NSAIDs may inhibit tendon cell migration and proliferation and impair tendon healing.[56] Nonetheless, these medications have analgesic properties that can be used for short periods to facilitate rehabilitation.[57,58]

There are few published data on the risks and benefits of using corticosteroid injections in treating Achilles tendinopathy, making their use controversial as well.[59–62] Peritendinous injection of corticosteroids has been associated with spontaneous rupture of the Achilles tendon based on individual case reports.[60,62,63] The few randomized controlled studies that have looked at local steroid use in Achilles tendinopathy show mixed results.[64–66] Due to the risk of spontaneous tendon rupture, the use of local corticosteroid injections is not recommended.[67]

Table 2
Pharmacologic treatment options for noninsertional Achilles tendinopathy

Intervention	Evidence	Conclusion
NSAIDs	One level I study	No definitive conclusion possible
Steroid injections	Two randomized controlled trials, several case series	Not recommended
PRP injection	One randomized controlled trials, several case series	No definitive conclusion possible
Sclerosis agents	Three randomized controlled trials, several case series	No definitive conclusion possible
High-volume injections	No randomized controlled trials, several case series	No definitive conclusion possible
Autologous blood injections	Two randomized controlled trials	No definitive conclusion possible

Additional injection therapy includes platelet-rich plasma (PRP), which is quickly gaining popularity in different areas of orthopedics. It is thought to enhance tendon healing by promoting the delivery of growth factors and cytokines that participate in tissue repair processes.[68–74] Early studies are also looking at how combination treatment with PRP and stem cells may serve as a promising therapeutic treatment of augmenting the tendon healing process. Results with stem cells are still variable and studies are preliminary[75,76]

The following two pharmacologic interventions target neovascularization, which is hypothesized as an indirect cause of pain in Achilles tendinopathy.[77] The ultrasound-guided injection of polidocanol (sclerosing agent) into peritendinous regions with high blood flow and nerves has been reported, in a small randomized controlled trial, to lead to pain relief and improved patient satisfaction.[78] Similarly, high-volume ultrasound-guided injections aim to prevent neovascularization through mechanical disruption of new vessels and their accompanying nerve supply.[78–83] Support of these treatments has not yet gained popularity because some less invasive eccentric exercises are also capable of decreasing neovascularization, thus providing pain relief to patients.[52,84]

COMBINATION THERAPIES

As discussed previously, there is a multitude of conservative treatment modalities offered to patients with Achilles tendinopathy; however, there is limited evidence supporting many of these measures. Some studies have looked at combination therapies, usually combining eccentric exercise with some other conservative therapy. A randomized controlled trial indicated significant improvement when extracorporeal shockwave therapy (ESWT) was combined with eccentric exercises compared with eccentric exercise alone.[85] It is suggested that ESWT works by disturbing the sensory nerve fibers and causing changes in the dorsal root ganglia, which may decrease the pain sensation.[86]

Similar to PRP, autologous blood injections are thought to stimulate growth and healing of the tendon and have been studied in combination with eccentric exercise. Combination treatment with autologous blood injections and eccentric exercise versus eccentric exercise alone indicated no additional benefit with the injections.[87–89]

SURGICAL TREATMENT OPTIONS

Like most orthopedic conditions, initial conservative treatment is the therapy of choice, but surgical intervention may be necessary once a patient has failed appropriate nonoperative treatment or the clinical situation remains unsatisfactory. In the case of Achilles tendinopathy, conservative treatment should be attempted for at least 6 months before surgery is recommended.[90] Approximately 24% to 45% of patients fail conservative management after 6 months.[49] Contraindications to surgery include arterial insufficiency, active skin infection, compromised soft tissue envelope, and select medical comorbidities that make a patient a high-risk surgical candidate.

There are a variety of described procedures for noninsertional Achilles tendinopathy, the goal of which is either to induce mild trauma to the degenerated tendon to initiate a healing response or to remove the diseased portion of tendon.[91] Considered likely the least invasive of the procedures, percutaneous longitudinal tenotomy is a technique described by Testa and colleagues,[92] where multiple ultrasound-guided and percutaneous incisions are made through the diseased portion of the Achilles tendon. This treatment has demonstrated successful results in 67% to 97% of patients, especially athletic patients, and worse outcomes in those individuals with more pervasive tendinopathy and paratendinopathy.[1,92,93] Many investigators believe that this surgery is indicated for mild-to-moderate, focal noninsertional Achilles tendinopathy. Percutaneous tenotomy should be considered for those individuals who have failed conservative treatment and are at risk for wound complications.[91]

Mini–open ultrasound and Doppler-guided scraping technique has been described by Alfredson and colleagues.[94] This method of tendon scraping targets the peritendinous tissues demonstrating ultrasound and Doppler-verified high blood flow on the ventral side of the Achilles tendon. The minimally invasive technique has demonstrated a high success rate at 1-year to 2-year follow-up.[95] Recent interest has focused on the role of the plantaris tendon in propagating Achilles tendinopathy. This muscle can become adherent to the medial aspect of the Achilles tendon, initiating an inflammatory response and localized tendinopathy. Studies have looked at combining the mini–open scraping with stripping of the plantaris tendon and its potential to improve tendon structure and reduce pain.[96,97] A few small studies, looking at release of the plantaris tendon, resulted in good outcomes with significant reduction in pain and improved function at 2 years.[98,99] To address the mechanical pathogenesis of this disease, a gastrocnemius recession has been proposed as a minimally invasive treatment option. Molund and colleagues[100] demonstrated promising short to midterm results, with excellent functional outcomes and pain resolution.

For moderate to severe tendinopathy, where perhaps adhesions may be difficult to remove with simple percutaneous procedures, open débridement may be necessary. This is a more extensive operation, where degenerative tendon tissue can be excised and the tendon should be inspected to confirm the extent of tendon involvement. The goals of open excision and repair of midsubstance Achilles tendinopathy are to excise fibrotic adhesions, remove degenerated nodules, identify and resect intratendinous lesions, and restore vascularity to remaining healthy tendinous tissue to help stimulate a healing response (**Figs. 4** and **5**). The ultimate goal is to restore function and strength of the Achilles tendon. The technique of endoscopic débridement for Achilles tendinopathy is also described with the potential advantage of minimally invasive surgery, faster recovery, and fewer postoperative complications. Although most series are small with short follow-up, results have overall been reported to be good.[101–103]

When at least 50% of the cross-sectional area of the tendon is composed of healthy fibers, then débridement and repair of the tendon via a technique known as tubularization is recommended.[91] When greater than 50% of the cross-sectional area of the

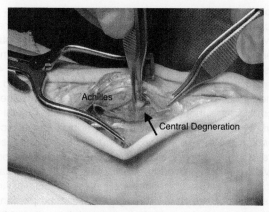

Fig. 4. Tendinopathic tissue: centralized degeneration with disorganized fiber bundles with a crab meat appearance.

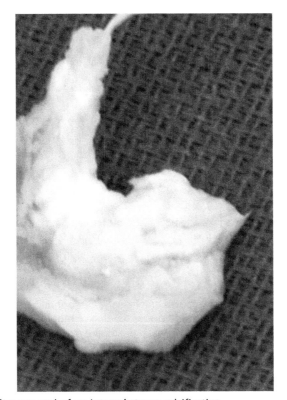

Fig. 5. Tissue after removal of an intrasubstance calcification.

tendon is diseased, however, then the tendon can be augmented after débridement and tubularization, with transfer of the flexor hallucis longus (FHL) muscle.[104] Open débridement has demonstrated favorable results.[105] The success of the procedure seems to be correlated with the duration of symptoms, with those patients whose symptoms have been present for a shorter period of time demonstrating improved surgical outcomes.[90,106] In general, most operative procedures for noninsertional Achilles tendinopathy are supported by fair evidence.

TREATMENT COMPLICATIONS

Treatment complications associated with surgery are not uncommon. Paavola and colleagues[107] reported an 11% postoperative complication rate in a large series of patients who underwent surgery for Achilles tendinopathy. The complications included wound necrosis in 3%, superficial infection in 2.5%, and sural nerve injury in 1% in addition to hematoma, seroma, deep venous thrombosis, and new partial ruptures.

Considerations for management of potential complications, such as sural nerve injury, include using a posteromedial incision and knowing the approximate nerve location at the lateral Achilles tendon border, 9.8 cm proximal to the calcaneal attachment.[108] Consider Strayer gastrocnemius recession, V-Y lengthening, turndown flap, or FHL transfer. A chevron excision of segments 2 cm to 3 cm can be performed and a biologic augmentation added[109] **(Fig. 6)**. Wound complications, including skin necrosis, wound dehiscence, and infections, are managed according to the size of the skin defect with either local wound care, myocutaneous flap, or free flap.

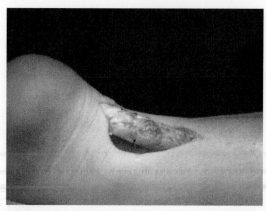

Fig. 6. Intraoperative photos of a patient with chronic tendinopathy requiring a 1.5-cm excision of the tendon. Final approximation of the tendon with an allograft augmentation (*arrow*) of the direct tendon repair.

SUMMARY

Achilles tendinopathy has been studied extensively. Current understanding of the etiology likely involves a combination of overuse leading to repetitive microtrauma, poor vascularity of the tissue, mechanical imbalances of the extremity, genetic predisposition, and a variety of metabolic factors. Histologic analysis has found abnormalities of the collagen fibers, cystic mucoid changes, tendolipomatosis, and calcific deposits as well as vascular changes. Biochemical and genetic analysis have revealed upregulation of matrix metalloproteinase 2, fibronectin subunit B, vascular endothelial growth factor, and mitogen-activated protein kinase p38 and down-regulation of matrix metalloproteinase 3 and decorin. The etiology, pathology, and optimal management have yet to be fully elucidated, however, and further high-quality investigation is warranted.

When diagnosed early, most patients respond to conservative measures; however, continuation of aggravating activities leads to chronic changes resistant to nonoperative treatment. There is research to support 12 weeks of eccentric exercise to reduce pain and decrease neovascularization, although the evidence is conflicting. Evidence to support the use of several other conservative modalities is limited, including anti-inflammatory medications, ultrasound, shock wave therapy, corticosteroid injections, PRP therapy, and prolotherapy with polidocanol. Operative interventions include percutaneous longitudinal tenotomies, minimally invasive tendon stripping, open tenosynovectomies, open débridement and tubularization, and tendon augmentation with FHL. There is fair evidence to recommend these procedures for Achilles tendinopathies recalcitrant to conservative measures.

Educating patients regarding symptomatic management and preventive measures may provide more benefit than leading them to believe that Achilles tendinopathy is completely curable. Future clarification of the underlying pathologic biology will allow for more effective management regimens and ultimately improve the success of both conservative and operative Achilles tendinopathy management.

REFERENCES

1. Courville XF, Coe MP, Hecht PJ. Current concepts review: noninsertional Achilles tendinopathy. Foot Ankle Int 2009;30(11):1132–42.

2. Roche AJ, Calder JF. Achilles tendinopathy: a review of the current concepts of treatment. Bone Joint J 2013;95(10):1299–307.
3. Almekinders LC, Temple JD. Etiology, diagnosis, and treatment of tendonitis: an analysis of the literature. Med Sci Sports Exerc 1998;30:1183–90.
4. Khan KM, Cook JL, Kannus P, et al. Time to abandon the "tendinitis" myth. BMJ 2002;324:626–7.
5. Waldecker U, Hofmann G, Drewitz S, et al. Epidemiologic investigation of 1394 feet: coincidence of hindfoot malalignmentand Achilles tendon disorders. Foot Ankle Surg 2012;18(2):119–23.
6. de Jonge S, van den Berg C, de Vos RJ, et al. Incidence of midportion Achilles tendinopathy in the general population. Br J Sports Med 2011;45:1026–8.
7. Lysholm J, Wiklander J. Injuries in runners. Am J Sports Med 1987;15:168–71.
8. Khan KM, Maffulli N. Tendinopathy: an Achilles' heel for athletes and clinicians. Clin J Sport Med 1998;8:151–4.
9. Sharma P, Maffulli N. Understanding and managing Achilles tendinopathy. Br J Hosp Med (Lond) 2006;67:64–7.
10. Van Middelkoop M, Kolkman J, Van Ochten J, et al. Prevalence and incidence of lower extremity injuries in male marathon runners. Scand J Med Sci Sports 2008; 18(2):140–4.
11. Kujala UM, Sarna S, Kaprio J, et al. Cumulative incidence of Achilles tendon rupture and tendinopathy in male former elite athletes. Clin J Sport Med 2005; 15(3):133–5.
12. Kannus P, Jozsa L. Histopathological changes preceding spontaneous rupture of a tendon. A controlled study of 891 patients. J Bone Joint Surg Am 1991; 73(10):1507–25.
13. Maffulli N, Longo UG, et al. Open management of achilles tendinopathy. Weisel SW, editor. Operative techniques in orthopedic surgery. 2011. p. 4443–6. Chapter 118.
14. Leadbetter WB. Cell-matrix response in tendon injury. Clin Sports Med 1992; 11(3):533–78.
15. Clements DB, Tunton JE, Smart GW, et al. Achilles tendinitis and peritendinitis. Etiology and treatment. Am J Sports Med 1984;12:179–86.
16. Komi PV, Fukashiro S, Järvinen M, et al. Biomechanical loading of achilles tendon during normal locomotion. Clin Sports Med 1992;11:521–31.
17. Kader D, Saxena A, Movin T, et al. Achilles tendinopathy: some aspects of basic science and clinical management. Br J Sports Med 2002;36(4):239–49.
18. Benazzo F, Maffulli N. An operative approach to achilles tendinopathy. Sports Med Arthrosc Rev 2000;8(1):96–101.
19. Lagergren C, Lindholm A. Vascular distribution in the achilles tendon; an angiographic and microangiographic study. Acta Chir Scand 1959;116(5–6): 491–5.
20. Ahmed IM, Lagopoulos M, McConnell P, et al. Blood supply of the achilles tendon. J Orthop Res 1998;16(5):591–6.
21. Astrom M, Westlin N. Blood flow in the human achilles tendon assessed by laser Doppler flowmetry. J Orthop Res 1994;12(2):246–52.
22. Niculescu V, Matusz P. The clinical importance of the calcaneal tendon vasculature (tendo calcaneus). Morphol Embryol (Bucur) 1988;34(1):5–8.
23. Carr AJ, Norris SH. The blood supply of the calcaneal tendon. J Bone Joint Surg Br 1989;71(1):100–1.
24. Chen TM, Rozen WM, Pan WR, et al. The arterial anatomy of the achilles tendon: anatomical study and clinical implications. Clin Anat 2009;22:377–85.

25. Astrom M, Westlin N. Blood flow in chronic achilles tendinopathy. Clin Orthop 1994;(308):166–72.
26. Holmes GB, Mann RA, et al. Epidemiological factors associated with rupture of the Achilles tendon. Contemp Orthop 1991;23:327–31.
27. Mokdad AH, Ford ES, Bowman BA, et al. Prevalence of obesity, diabetes, and obesity-related health risk factors. JAMA 2003;289(1):76–9.
28. Williams IL, Wheatcroft SB, Shah AM, et al. Obesity, atherosclerosis and the vascular endothelium: mechanisms of reduced nitric oxide bioavailability in obese humans. Int J Obes Relat Metab Disord 2002;26(6):754–64.
29. Holmes GB, Lin J. Etiologic factors associated with symptomatic achilles tendinopathy. Foot Ankle Int 2006;27(11):952–9.
30. Grant WP, Sullivan R, Sonenshine DE, et al. Electron microscopic investigation of the effects of diabetes mellitus on the Achilles tendon. J Foot Ankle Surg 1997; 36(4):272–8.
31. Batista F, Nery C, Pinzur M, et al. Achilles tendinopathy in diabetes mellitus. Foot Ankle Int 2008;29(5):498–501.
32. Strocchi R, De Pasquale V, Guizzardi S, et al. Human achilles tendon: morphological and morphometric variations as a function of age. Foot Ankle 1991;12(2): 100–4.
33. Kirchgesner T, Larbi A, Omoumi P, et al. Drug-induced tendinopathy: from physiology to clinical applications. Joint Bone Spine 2014;81(6):485–92.
34. Kvist M. Achilles tendon injuries in athletes. Ann Chir Gynaecol 1991;80(2): 188–201.
35. Nigg BM. The role of impact forces and foot pronation: a new paradigm. Clin J Sport Med 2001;11(1):2–9.
36. Kannus P. Etiology and pathophysiology of chronic tendon disorders in sports. Scand J Med Sci Sports 1997;7(2):78–85.
37. Jozsa L, Kannus P. Human tendon: anatomy, physiology and pathology. Champaign (IL): Human Kinetics; 1997.
38. Alfredson H, Lorentzon M, Bäckman S, et al. cDNA-arrays and real-time quantitative PCR techniques in the investigation of chronic Achilles tendinosis. J Orthop Res 2003;21:970–5.
39. Maffulli N. Re: etiologic factors associated with symptomatic achilles tendinopathy. Foot Ankle Int 2007;28(5):660–1.
40. Maffulli N, Kader D. Tendinopathy of tendo Achilles. J Bone Joint Surg Br 2002; 84(1):1–8.
41. Maffulli N, Kenward MG, Testa V, et al. Clinical diagnosis of achilles tendinopathy with tendinosis. Clin J Sport Med 2003;13(1):11–5.
42. Maffulli N, Khan KM, Puddu G, et al. Overuse tendon conditions: time to change a confusing terminology. Arthroscopy 1998;14(8):840–3.
43. Maffulli N, Sharma P, Luscombe KL, et al. Achilles tendinopathy: aetiology and management. J R Soc Med 2004;97(1):472–6.
44. Alfredson H, Cook J. A treatment algorithm for managing Achilles tendinopathy: new treatment options. Br J Sports Med 2007;41(4):211–6.
45. Alfredson H, Lorentzon R. Chronic achilles tendinosis: recommendations for treatment and prevention. Sports Med 2000;29:135–46.
46. Rompe J, Nafe B, Furia JP, et al. Eccentric loading, shock wave treatment, or a wait-and-see policy for tendinopathy of the main body of teno Achillitis: a randomized controlled trial. Am J Sports Med 2007;35(3):374–83.
47. Rompe JD, Furia JP, Maffulli N, et al. Mid-portion achilles tendinopathy current options for treatment. Disabil Rehabil 2008;30(20–22):1666–76.

48. Leadbetter WB. Tendon overuse injuries. Diagnosis and treatment. In: Renstrom PAFH, editor. Sport injuries: basic principles of prevention and care. Boston: Blackwell Scientific Publications; 1993. p. 449–76.
49. Paavola M, Kannus P, Paakkala T, et al. Long-term prognosis of patients with achilles tendinopathy: an observational 8-year follow-up study. Am J Sports Med 2000;28:634–42.
50. Alfredson H, Pietila T, Jonsson P, et al. Heavy-load eccentric calf muscle training for the treatment of chronic Achilles tendinosis. Am J Sports Med 1998;26: 360–6.
51. Magnussen RA, Dunn WR, Thomson AB, et al. Nonoperative treatment of mid-portion Achilles tendinopathy: a systematic review. Clin J Sport Med 2009; 19(1):54–64.
52. Ohberg L, Alfredson H. Effects on neovascularisation behind the good results with eccentric training in chronic mid-portion achilles tendinosis? Knee Surg Sports Traumatol Arthrosc 2004;12(5):465–70.
53. Mayer F, Hirschmuller A. Effects of short-term treatment strategies over 4 weeks in Achilles tendinopathy. Br J Sports Med 2007;41:e6.
54. de Vos RJ, Weir A, Visser RJ, et al. The additional value of a night splint to eccentric exercises in chronic midportion Achilles tendinopathy: a randomised controlled trial. Br J Sports Med 2007;41:e5.
55. de Jonge S, de Vos RJ, Van Schie HT, et al. One-year follow-up of a randomised controlled trial on added splinting to eccentric exercises in chronic midportion Achilles tendinopathy. Br J Sports Med 2010;44:673–7.
56. Tsai WC, Hsu CC, Chou SW, et al. Effects of celecoxib on migration, proliferation and collagen expression of tendon cells. Connect Tissue Res 2007;48(1):46–51.
57. Sandmeier R, Renström PA. Diagnosis and treatment of chronic tendon disorders in sports. Scand J Med Sci Sports 1997;7:96–106.
58. Leadbetter WB. Anti-inflammatory therapy and sports injury: the role of non-steroidal drugs and corticosteroid injection. Clin Sports Med 1995;14: 353–410.
59. Shrier I, Matheson GO, Kohl HW. Achilles tendonitis: are corticosteroid injections useful or harmful? Clin J Sport Med 1996;6:245–50.
60. Fredberg U. Local corticosteroid injection in sport: review of literature and guidelines for treatment. Scand J Med Sci Sports 1997;7:131–9.
61. Speed CA. Fortnightly review: corticosteroid injections in tendon lesions. BMJ 2001;323:382–6.
62. Paavola M, Kannus P, Järvinen TAH, et al. Tendon healing: adverse role of steroid injection—myth or reality. Foot Ankle Clin 2002;7:501–13.
63. Gill SS, Gelbke MK, Mattson SL, et al. Fluoroscopically guided low-volume peritendinous corticosteroid injection for Achilles tendinopathy. A safety study. J Bone Joint Surg Am 2004;86-A(4):802–6.
64. DaCruz DJ, Geeson M, Allen MJ, et al. Achilles paratendonitis: an evaluation of steroid injection. Br J Sports Med 1988;22:64–5.
65. Neeter C, Thomee R, Silbernagel KG, et al. Iontophoresis with or without dexamethasone in the treatment of acute Achilles tendon pain. Scand J Med Sci Sports 2003;13:376–82.
66. Fredberg U, Bolvig L, Pfeiffer-Jensen M, et al. Ultrasonography as a tool for diagnosis, guidance of local steroid injection and, together with pressure algometry, monitoring of the treatment of athletes with chronic jumper's knee and Achilles tendonitis: a randomized, double-blind, placebo-controlled study. Scand J Rheumatol 2004;33:94–101.

67. Coombes BK. Efficacy and safety of corticosteroid injections and other injections for management of tendinopathy: a systematic review of randomised controlled trials. Lancet 2010;376(9754):1751–67.

68. Foster TE, Puskas BL, Mandelbaum BR, et al. Platelet-rich plasma: from basic science to clinical applications. Am J Sports Med 2009;37:2259–72.

69. de Mos M, van der Windt AE, Jahr H, et al. Can platelet-rich plasma enhance tendon repair? A cell culture study. Am J Sports Med 2008;36:1171–8.

70. Sinnott C, White HM, et al. Autologous blood and platelet rich plasma injections in the treatment of achilles tendinopathy: a critically appraised topic. J Sport Rehabil 2016;24:1–15.

71. de Jonge S, de Vos RJ, Weir A, et al. One-year follow-up of platelet-rich plasma treatment in chronic Achilles tendinopathy: a double-blind randomized placebo-controlled trial. Am J Sports Med 2011;39:1623–9.

72. De Vos RJ, Weir A, Tol JL, et al. No effects of PRP on ultrasonographic tendon structure and neovascularisation in chronic midportion Achilles tendinopathy. Br J Sports Med 2011;45:387–92.

73. de Vos RJ, Weir A, van Schie HT, et al. Platelet-rich plasma injection for chronic Achilles tendinopathy: a randomized controlled trial. JAMA 2010;303:144–9.

74. Sadoghi P, Rosso C, Valderrabano V, et al. The role of platelets in the treatment of achilles tendon injuries. J Orthop Res 2013;31:111–8.

75. Chiou G, Crowe C, McGoldrick R, et al. Optimization of an injectable tendon hydrogel: the effects of platelet rich plasma and adipose-derived stem cells on tendon healing in vivo. Tissue Eng Part A 2015;21(9–10):1579–86.

76. Ahmad Z, Wardale K, Brooks R, et al. Exploring the application of stem cells in tendon repair and regeneration. Arthroscopy 2012;28(7):1018–29.

77. Ohberg L, Lorentzon R, Alfredson H. Neovascularisation in Achilles tendons with painful tendinosis but not in normal tendons: an ultrasonographic investigation. Knee Surg Sports Traumatol Arthrosc 2001;9:233–8.

78. Alfredson H, Lorentzon R. Sclerosing polidocanol injections of small vessels to treat the chronic painful tendon. Cardiovasc Hematol Agents Med Chem 2007;5:97–100.

79. Alfredson H, Ohberg L. Sclerosing injections to areas of neo-vascularisation reduce pain in chronic Achilles tendinopathy: a double-blind randomised controlled trial. Knee Surg Sports Traumatol Arthrosc 2005;13:338–44.

80. Lind B, Ohberg L, Alfredson H. Sclerosing polidocanol injections in mid-portion Achilles tendinosis: remaining good clinical results and decreased tendon thickness at 2-year follow-up. Knee Surg Sports Traumatol Arthrosc 2006;14: 1327–32.

81. Chan O, O'Dowd D, Padhiar N, et al. High volume image guided injections in chronic Achilles tendinopathy. Disabil Rehabil 2008;30:1697–708.

82. Maffulli N, Spiezia F, Longo UG, et al. High volume image guided injections for the management of chronic tendinopathy of the main body of the Achilles tendon. Phys Ther Sport 2013;14(3):163–7.

83. Humphrey J, Chan O, Crisp T, et al. The short-term effects of high volume image guided injections in resistant non-insertional Achilles tendinopathy. J Sci Med Sport 2010;13:295–8.

84. Ohberg L, Lorentzon R, Alfredson H. Eccentric training in patients with chronic Achilles tendinosis: normalised tendon structure and decreased thickness at follow up. Br J Sports Med 2004;38:8–11.

85. Rompe JD, Furia J, Maffulli N. Eccentric loading versus eccentric loading plus shock-wave treatment for midportion achilles tendinopathy: a randomized controlled trial. Am J Sports Med 2009;37:463–70.

86. Mani-Babu S, Morrissey D, Waugh C, et al. The effectiveness of extracorporeal shock wave therapy in lower limb tendinopathy: a systematic review. Am J Sports Med 2015;42(3):752–61.
87. de Vos RJ, van Veldhoven PL, Moen MH, et al. Autologous growth factor injections in chronic tendinopathy: a systematic review. Br Med Bull 2010;95:63–77.
88. Bell KJ, Fulcher ML, Rowlands DS, et al. Impact of autologous blood injections in treatment of mid-portion Achilles tendinopathy: double blind randomized controlled trial. BMJ 2013;346:f2310.
89. Pearson J, Rowlands D, Highet R. Autologous blood injection to treat Achilles tendinopathy? A randomized controlled trial. J Sport Rehabil 2012;21(3): 218–24.
90. Johnston E, Scranton P Jr, Pfeffer GB, et al. Chronic disorders of the Achilles tendon: results of conservative and surgical treatments. Foot Ankle Int 1997; 18(9):570–4.
91. Scott AT, Le IL, Easley ME, et al. Surgical strategies: noninsertional Achilles tendinopathy. Foot Ankle Int 2008;29(7):759–71.
92. Testa V, Capasso G, Benazzo F, et al. Management of Achilles tendinopathy by ultrasound-guided percutaneous tenotomy. Med Sci Sports Exerc 2002;34(4): 573–80.
93. Maffulli N, Testa V, Capasso G, et al. Results of percutaneous longitudinal tenotomy for Achilles tendinopathy in middle- and long-distance runners. Am J Sports Med 1997;25(6):835–40.
94. Alfredson H, Ohberg L, Zeisig E, et al. Treatment of midportion Achilles tendinosis: similar clinical results with US and CD-guided surgery outside the tendon and sclerosing polidocanol injections. Knee Surg Sports Traumatol Arthrosc 2007;15:1504–9.
95. Alfredson H. Ultrasound and Doppler-guided mini-surgery to treat mid-portion Achilles tendinosis: results of a large material and a randomised study comparing two scraping techniques. Br J Sports Med 2011;45:407–10.
96. van Sterkenburg MN, Kerkhoffs GM, Kleipool RP, et al. The plantaris tendon and a potential role in mid-portion Achilles tendinopathy: an observational anatomical study. J Anat 2011;218:336–41.
97. Lintz F, Higgs A, Millett M, et al. The role of plantaris longus in achilles tendinopathy: a biomechanical study. Foot Ankle Surg 2011;17:252–5.
98. van Sterkenburg MN, Kerkhoffs GM, van Dijk CN, et al. Good outcome after stripping the plantaris tendon in patients with chronic mid-portion Achilles tendinopathy. Knee Surg Sports Traumatol Arthrosc 2011;19:1362–6.
99. Pearce CJ, Carmichael J, Calder JD, et al. Achilles tendinoscopy and plantaris tendon release and division in the treatment of non-insertional Achilles tendinopathy. Foot Ankle Surg 2012;18:124–7.
100. Molund M, Lapinskas SR, Nilsen FA, et al. Clinical and functional outcomes of gastrocnemius recession for chronic achilles tendinopathy. Foot Ankle Int 2016;37(10):1091–7.
101. Maquirriain J. Surgical treatment of chronic Achilles tendinopathy: long-term results of the endoscopic technique. J Foot Ankle Surg 2013;52:451–5.
102. Maquirriain J, Ayerza M, Costa-Paz M, et al. Endoscopic surgery in chronic achillles tendinopathies; a preliminary report. Arthroscopy 2002;18: 298–303.
103. Lui T. Treatment of chronic noninsertional Achilles tendinopathy with endoscopic Achilles tendon debridement and flexor hallucis longus transfer. Foot Ankle Spec 2012;3:195–200.

104. Wapner KL, Pavlock GS, Hecht PJ, et al. Repair of chronic Achilles tendon rupture with flexor hallucis longus tendon transfer. Foot Ankle 1993;14:443–9.

105. Leach RE, Schepsis AA, Takai H, et al. Long-term results of surgical management of Achilles tendinitis in runners. Clin Orthop Relat Res 1992;282:208–12.

106. Maffulli N, Binfield PM, Moore D, et al. Surgical decompression of chronic central core lesions of the Achilles tendon. Am J Sports Med 1999;27(6):747–52.

107. Paavola M, Orava S, Leppilahti J, et al. Chronic Achilles tendon overuse injury: complications after surgical treatment. An analysis of 432 consecutive patients. Am J Sports Med 2000;28(1):77–82.

108. Webb J, Niemann M, Lanz R, et al. Anatomy of the sural nerve and its relation to the Achilles tendon. Foot Ankle Int 2000;21:475–7.

100. Giza E, Frizzell L, Farac R, et al. Augmented tendon Achilles repair using a tissue reinforcement scaffold: a biomechanical study. Foot Ankle Int 2011;32(5): 545–9.

Insertional Tendinopathy of the Achilles

Debridement, Primary Repair, and When to Augment

Rachel J. Shakked, MD, Steven M. Raikin, MD*

KEYWORDS

- Enthesopathy • Haglund deformity • Calcific tendonitis
- Flexor hallucis longus tendon transfer

KEY POINTS

- Achilles tendinopathy is considered by most to be a degenerative enthesopathy with increased vascularity; however, some literature suggests an inflammatory process as well.
- Nonsurgical management may consist of eccentric training, although the success rate of this technique may not be as high as when utilized for midsubstance Achilles tendinopathy.
- Surgical treatment involves tendon debridement via a medial, midline, or lateral approach with variable detachment of the tendon insertion.
- Flexor hallucis longus tendon transfer via a single approach can help to augment the repair; studies remain equivocal on the clinical benefit of this procedure.
- Tendon repair after detachment is best accomplished with at least 2 suture anchors; a second row of anchors may improve the tendon footprint but has not been shown to be significantly beneficial in clinical studies.

BACKGROUND

Insertional Achilles tendinopathy is an enthesopathy involving the distal portion of the Achilles tendon and its insertion into the posterior calcaneal tuberosity. Insertional tendinopathy occurs frequently in runners and other athletes, but also is commonly seen in the older, heavier population.[1–3] An association between systemic diseases such as hypertension and diabetes with Achilles tendinopathy has also been demonstrated.[3] The pathogenesis is not fully understood but is considered to be degenerative and

Disclosure: The authors have nothing to disclose.
Foot and Ankle Service, Rothman Institute at Jefferson, Sidney Kimmel Medical College, 925 Chestnut Street, 5th Floor, Philadelphia, PA 19107, USA
* Corresponding author.
E-mail address: Steven.Raikin@rothmaninstitute.com

associated with increasing age, increased vascularity, and overuse.[4–6] This is not thought to be an inflammatory tendonitis with histopathology demonstrating disorganized collagen, abnormal neovascularization, and mucoid degeneration.[7] However, there may be a combination of degenerative and inflammatory changes that lead to Achilles tendinopathy. Recent studies have demonstrated inflammatory cells in areas of Achilles tendinopathy.[8,9] A biopsy study of 50 cases of Achilles tendinopathy compared with 15 healthy tendons demonstrated greater numbers of macrophages and endothelial cells in the study group compared with the control.[10] Furthermore, better outcomes at final follow-up were seen in patients who had iron positive hemosiderophages at initial biopsy, a sign of an inflammatory response. Insertional Achilles tendinopathy tends to involve the anterior part of the tendon, although the highest strain on biomechanical testing is actually posterior.[11] There is a high association between insertional Achilles tendinopathy and an enlarged or prominent superior posterolateral calcaneal tuberosity termed a Haglund deformity.[12] While a Haglund deformity may be present in the asymptomatic population, it is postulated that the anterior Achilles insertion rubs against the bony prominence, particularly when associated with a tight or contracted gastroc-soleus-Achilles myotendinous complex, resulting in local damage to the tendon and even intratendinous longitudinal tears at the insertion.

Nicholson and colleagues[13] described a system to predict potential success of nonoperative treatment of insertional Achilles tendinosis depending on degree of involvement of the tendon. Type I involvement (tendon thickening < 8 mm with nonuniform intramural splits) had the greatest chance of success (87.5%), while greater involvement (types II and III) had 90% and 70% failure rates, respectively. However, Lu and colleagues[14] found no correlation between the size of the Haglund process and the development of symptoms or outcome of treatment.

There is additionally a high proportion of patients who have calcification or spurs at the insertion of the Achilles into the calcaneus. The pathophysiology of these painful calcifications and bone spurs continues to be evaluated. Some have theorized that cartilage-like changes that typically occur on the anterior side of the tendon later undergo intratendinous bone formation via enchondral ossification.[7] Others theorize that bone spurs occur dorsally as an adaptive process to provide more surface area, not as a result of microtears or tendon trauma.[15]

CLINICAL PRESENTATION AND EVALUATION

Patients typically present with pain and swelling posterior to the tendon that most commonly has a lateral focus. Retrocalcaneal bursitis may occur concomitantly and may be related to inflammation about the Haglund deformity.[4] Symptoms usually occur with activity, but can occur at all times as the disease progresses. Clinically there is local tenderness at the Achilles insertion, and the Haglund deformity is prominently felt at the superior aspect of the posterolateral calcaneal tuberosity. The Achilles tendon is usually tight or contracted, and a Silfverskiold test should be performed to differentiate gastrocnemius versus soleus involvement. This is done by evaluating ankle dorsiflexion with the knee flexed and extended. If the ankle dorsiflexion increases with knee flexion, this suggests predominant gastrocnemius muscle contracture, compared with soleus or combined contracture if there is no difference in ankle dorsiflexion with the knee flexed or extended.

Radiographic assessment is undertaken with a weight-bearing lateral radiograph. This may demonstrate intratendinous calcification, insertional spurring, and/or a prominent Haglund deformity (**Fig. 1**). Two common radiographic measurements are used to evaluate the severity of the Haglund deformity. The Fowler and Philip

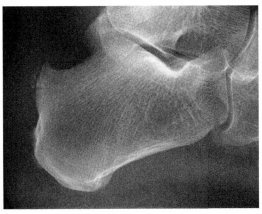

Fig. 1. Standing lateral radiograph demonstrating a prominent Haglund deformity and calcific deposits within the Achilles tendon substance.

posterior calcaneal angle is the angle subtended between a line along the plantar surface of the calcaneal tuberosity and a line tangent to the most prominent points along the posterior aspect of the tuberosity (**Fig. 2**).[16] An angle greater than 75° is considered abnormal. The parallel pitch lines (PPLs) described by Pavlov and colleagues[17] refer to a line drawn along the most prominent portions of the plantar surface of the calcaneal tuberosity and a parallel line starting at the most posterior aspect of the subtalar posterior facet joint (**Fig. 3**). A normal Haglund process is at or below the superior line, whereas an abnormal process extends beyond the superior line and is considered a positive PPL (see **Fig. 3**). This has been shown to significantly correlate with clinical symptoms.[17] MRI is useful to assess the involvement of the Achilles tendon. Tendon abnormalities may be seen in asymptomatic patients, although bone marrow edema near the tendon insertion is almost always associated with symptoms.[18] MRI can also predict success of nonoperative treatment; with significant intrasubstance signal abnormalities, there is a reduced chance of successful nonsurgical treatment (**Fig. 4**).[13] Ultrasound may also be a useful and less expensive modality to evaluate the quality of the tendon, although it is operator-dependent. When compared to intraoperative findings, similar information is gleaned from MRI and ultrasound.[19]

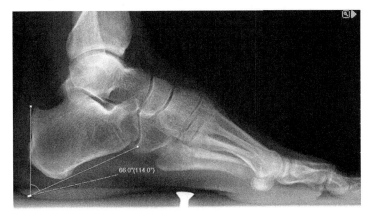

Fig. 2. Standing lateral radiograph demonstrating the Fowler and Philip posterior calcaneal angle.

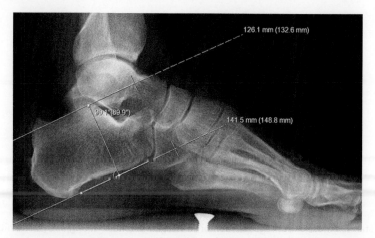

Fig. 3. Standing lateral radiograph demonstrating Pavlov parallel pitch lines. The Haglund process extends above the drawn line, indicating a positive parallel pitch line.

NONSURGICAL MANAGEMENT

Most agree that a course of nonsurgical treatment of 3 to 6 months is appropriate prior to considering surgical treatment. Activity modification and rest in addition to heel lifts and/or boot immobilization can help alleviate symptoms. Physical therapy with a focus on eccentric training has shown success in several studies, although it tends to work better for noninsertional tendinopathy with an 89% success rate.[20] However, utilizing a modified eccentric strengthening protocol that eliminates dorsiflexion beyond neutral, clinical improvement was shown in 67% of patients.[21] Extracorporeal shock

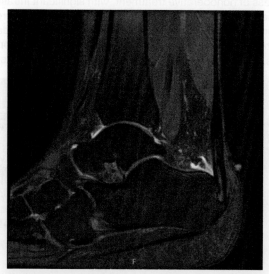

Fig. 4. Sagittal T2-weighted MRI image demonstrating increased signal within the substance of the Achilles tendon at its insertion. Increased signal is also seen in the retrocalcaneal bursa.

wave therapy may be a useful modality that has been shown to fare better than eccentric training in clinical studies.[22] No studies have evaluated the effects of platelet reduced plasma or steroid injections on insertional Achilles tendinopathy.

SURGICAL MANAGEMENT
Approaches

Surgical treatment of insertional Achilles tendinopathy is indicated in symptomatic patients who have failed nonsurgical treatment for a period of 3 to 6 months. There are multiple surgical approaches and techniques that have shown clinical success. In a retrospective case series of 35 patients, tendon debridement via a lateral approach was associated with complete or significant relief of symptoms in 90% of patients.[23] Another study evaluating the lateral approach with 80% tendon detachment, debridement, and 2-suture anchor repair demonstrated improved American Orthopedic Foot and Ankle Society (AOFAS) hindfoot scores at 1 year from 44 to 87, visual analog scale (VAS) from 7.2 to 1.7, and Short Form (SF) 36 scores.

A lateral or medial approach to the tendon avoids the midline watershed region and can minimize scar sensitivity with shoewear, but may not provide complete access to the tendon or allow for thorough debridement. Patients with calcific tendinopathy operatively treated with a posterolateral approach and minimal tendon detachment were less satisfied than those without calcific tendinopathy and had greater pain and shoe restrictions.[24] Partial tendon detachment in another study utilizing a medial approach and a horizontal limb distal to the tendon insertion demonstrated greater than 90% patient satisfaction without reservations.[25] Sixteen of 21 patients (76%) reported excellent or good outcomes after tendon debridement via a medial approach.[26] A variable percentage of the tendon was detached, and greater numbers of suture anchors were used accordingly for repair. Patients were pain-free after about 12 months, although 25% were unable to return to their previous level of activity.[26]

Despite reasonable outcomes after a medial or lateral approach, some advocate for a midline posterior approach with tendon splitting in order to adequately debride the tendinotic regions. In a series of 40 patients who underwent tendon-splitting Achilles and bony process debridement, patients demonstrated significant improvement in symptoms based on AOFAS hindfoot scores, Foot and Ankle Outcome Score (FAOS), pain scores, and SF-12 scores at 16 months postoperatively.[27] The tendon was repaired in a variety of ways including single anchor, double anchor, or double row constructs. Patients with at least a 2-anchor repair were noted to have significantly better functional scores than those patients with a single anchor. There was also a nonsignificant but continued trend toward improved outcomes after double-row repair. Although patients improved, the overall functional scores at final follow-up were slightly lower than seen in other studies.[28–30] This was explained by the relatively short time period of follow-up, but outcomes were also more similar among the subgroup of patients with 2-anchor repair. Excellent outcomes were achieved in another study utilizing a central splitting approach with 2-anchor repair in 39 patients.[30] AOFAS scores were over 90 and VAS under 15 at 1-year follow-up with central splitting approach and 2 anchor repair in 39 patients. A portion of this group underwent flexor hallucis longus (FHL) transfer, but outcomes were similar among groups.

Long-term data also support good outcomes with the central splitting approach. In a retrospective series of 27 patients, a central-splitting approach was performed with up to 70% elevation of the tendon.[28] The tendon was debrided up to 50% of its thickness, and calcifications were removed. The distal spur and Haglund deformity were excised, and the tendon was repaired with 2 suture anchors. Pain resolution occurred at an average of 5.7 months. Recurrent calcification occurred in 50% (11 of 22) of cases who returned at 4-year follow-up. No strength deficit was observed on isokinetic testing of ankle plantarflexion. At 7-year follow-up, 96% of patients (22 of 23) were completely pain-free and highly satisfied with surgery.

Tendon Reattachment

Two-anchor repair in a single row is a common construct seen in the recent Achilles tendinopathy literature (**Fig. 5**). New attention is focused on the double-row suture anchor construct, which may be beneficial because of the increased footprint area of the tendon on the calcaneal tuberosity. The increased fixation may allow for earlier weight-bearing and rehabilitation to expedite the recovery process. Several biomechanical studies have evaluated the benefit of a double-row construct versus single-row construct. One study with industry funding demonstrated greater peak load to failure with a double-row construct compared with a single-row construct.[31] However, another study without industry funding failed to show a difference in load to failure between single- and double-row constructs.[32] Another technique utilizes a suture button in addition to double-row fixation.[33] Peak load to failure measured 391 N compared with 239 N in the double-row repair without augmentation. In a previous study, the peak load to failure of the double-row repair without a suture button measured 434 N, although load to failure was tested at different speeds among these studies.[31] A knotless suture construct is theoretically optimal when repairing the Achilles in order to avoid prominent knots and skin irritation in an area that lacks a robust soft tissue

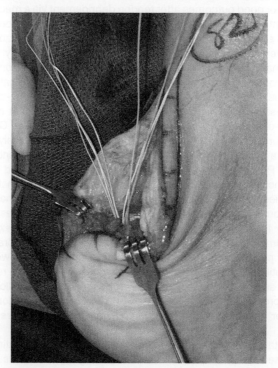

Fig. 5. Intraoperative photograph demonstrating position of anchor placement for 2-anchor, single-row tendon repair.

sleeve. The knotless double-row repair has been shown to have a lower peak load to failure than the knotted version, but this may be due to the larger perforation in the tendon due to the thick, braided suture variety associated with this procedure.[34] A rip stop suture placed distal to the suture may prevent propagation of the tendon perforation and improve peak load to failure, but requires additional investigation.

None of these repairs can tolerate normal peak Achilles tendon forces, which average 1430 N with normal walking.[35] However, stronger repairs may theoretically allow for a more aggressive rehabilitation program. Aside from biomechanical studies that suggest the benefit of a double-row repair, clinical outcomes may trend better when compared with a single- or double-anchor repair. Statistically significant functional improvement was shown when comparing double-anchor or double-row repair with single-anchor repair.[27]

Tendon Augmentation

The FHL tendon can be transferred to the calcaneal tuberosity for additional structural support after debriding the Achilles tendon. The FHL is a flexor tendon that crosses the ankle and is therefore in-phase with the Achilles. The muscle belly is relatively low-lying and is thought to optimize the healing response and perfuse the healing Achilles tendon.[36–39] It is generally accepted that FHL transfer is indicated in cases of greater than 50% tendon debridement in order to reduce the risk of tendon avulsion.[40] There should also be a low threshold to perform FHL transfer in the older, heavier patient.[41–43] Although there are a variety of methods of harvest and fixation of the tendon graft, the single-incision technique affords adequate access to the tendon and high satisfaction rates.[41–45] Nonetheless, the clinical benefit of FHL transfer has recently come into question after a prospective, randomized study in 39 patients over age 50 years failed to show a significant functional benefit.[30] Although not a validated measure, 1-year AOFAS scores improved from 57 to 92 points in the control group and 61 to 92 points in the FHL transfer group. The 1-year VAS score improved from 68 to 15 points in the control group and 64 to 10 points in the experimental group. FHL transfer did improve plantarflexion strength without causing any significant hallux plantarflexion weakness. Although not statistically significant, there was a trend toward greater wound healing issues in patients who underwent FHL transfer compared with the control group.

Haglund Excision

The Haglund deformity is thought to irritate the tendon in cases of insertional tendinopathy, and decompression of any bony impingement on the tendon is a routine component of surgical debridement for tendinopathy. However, some authors suggest that the Haglund deformity plays less of a role in the process than previously thought; a radiographic study of 48 heels with insertional Achilles tendinopathy versus 50 asymptomatic heels failed to demonstrate a statistical difference in measurements of the Haglund deformity.[12] Sixteen of 21 patients in another case series were found to have excellent or good outcomes after tendon debridement without excision of the Haglund deformity.[26]

A recent study has described utilizing a low-speed high-torque burr to perform a limited open dorsal closing wedge osteotomy of the calcaneus to treat Haglund exostosis in athletes.[46] The osteotomy, initially described by Zadek,[47] was used in 52 patients with an average return to sport at 20 weeks, and 96% good or excellent results at 3 years. Only limited studies are published on this procedure, and further investigation is required at this point.

SENIOR AUTHOR'S PREFERRED SURGICAL TECHNIQUE

The patient is positioned in a prone position on a well-padded chest roll (**Fig. 6**). A thigh tourniquet is utilized. If there is concern that the entire insertion may need to be released in order to adequately debride the abnormal portion of the tendon, both limbs should be prepared and draped to allow the resting tension of the repair to match that of the normal limb.

An 8 cm longitudinal midline incision is made over the posterior aspect of the Achilles tendon, extending down over the Haglund exostosis and the insertion of the spur to the glabrous skin junction at the heel (**Fig. 7**). The incision is made full-thickness down to the level of the paratenon to ensure vascular skin flaps. The paratenon is then reflected off the distal Achilles tendon (**Fig. 8**).

The distal Achilles tendon is evaluated clinically by palpation for abnormal thickening and intrasubstance ossification. The tendon is split longitudinally down the center into medial and lateral portions, down to the insertion into the calcaneus (**Fig. 9**). Any intratendinous ossifications are excised. The splitting of the tendon allows evaluation of the entire anterior portion of the tendon for tendinotic damage (**Fig. 10**). The tendinotic portion of the tendon loses its striated shiny appearance and is often referred to as resembling fish flesh. This tendinotic tissue must all be excised until healthy tendinous tissue is seen (**Fig. 11**). This may require 70% or more of the tendon to be elevated off the bony insertion for adequate visualization and debridement. Any intrasubstance tears are debrided and excised.

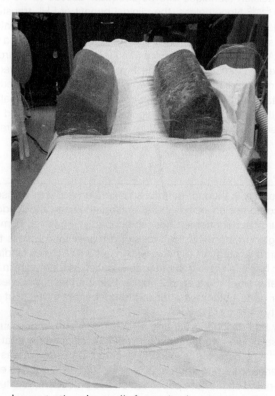

Fig. 6. Bed set-up demonstrating chest rolls for optimal patient position.

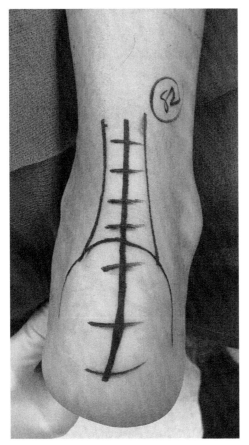

Fig. 7. Landmarks drawn on skin, including calcaneal tuberosity and Achilles tendon, as well as the planned midline incision.

Once the tendon has been split and reflected, the Haglund exostosis can be seen. This, together with any insertional spurs, are removed with an osteotome or sagittal saw (**Fig. 12**A, B). It is important to resect an adequate amount of bone from the posterior superior calcaneal tuberosity to ensure that the insertion reattachment of the Achilles tendon is fully decompressed. The resection should start distal to the insertional spur and Haglund posteriorly, and extend to exit dorsally and anteriorly, proximal to the posterior aspect of the subtalar joint posterior facet (see **Fig. 12**B).

If there are severe tendinotic changes at the insertion requiring that more than 50% of the distal tendinous insertion be excised, an FHL transfer is recommended to augment the repair. This additionally may be indicated for obese and older patients who may benefit from the augmented strength of the FHL muscle. The FHL muscle and tendon lie in the deep posterior compartment of the leg, immediately anterior to the Kager fat pad situated anterior to the Achilles tendon. The deep compartment fascia is incised longitudinally over the midline, and the FHL is easily identified by its distal muscle belly, which is visualized at the level of the posterior ankle joint (**Fig. 13**). The tibial nerve lies just medial to the FHL tendon, so all dissection must be performed over the lateral aspect of the FHL to prevent inadvertent nerve injury. The sheath of the FHL tendon

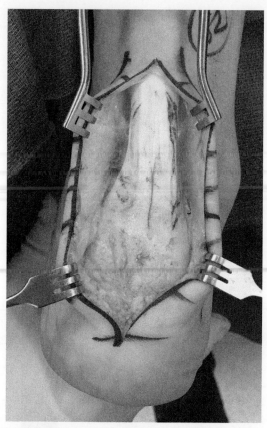

Fig. 8. The skin and paratenon have been elevated to expose the Achilles tendon insertion, which is thickened and calcified.

is released as the tendon runs medial to the posterior talar process and behind the medial malleolus. Once appropriate a length of tendon (5-6 cm) is obtained, the tendon is transected and retracted out of the incision region. Always cut the FHL from medial to lateral to prevent injury to the tibial nerve. A whip stitch using #0 braided absorbable suture is run through the distal FHL tendon, and the tendon diameter is measured. A Beath pin is then drilled from dorsal to plantar through the posterior calcaneus just anterior to the Achilles tendon insertion (**Fig. 14**A, B). A matching diameter bone tunnel is then drilled over the Beath pin using sized reamers. The #0 suture in the FHL is then threaded through the eyelet of the Beath pin, which is then used to pull the suture through the bottom of the heel. The foot is held in 30° of plantarflexion while the FHL tendon is maximally tensioned by pulling the suture, delivering the tendon into the bone tunnel (**Fig. 15**). The FHL will usually stretch out during recovery and is rarely tensioned too tightly. The screw is inserted while maximum tension is applied to the FHL tendon. A bioabsorbable interference screw 1 mm larger than the bone tunnel is utilized so as to obtain optimal fixation in the cancellous bone of the calcaneus.

Once this is completed, the Achilles tendon is reattached to the calcaneus. The senior author's preference is to use a single row of 2 3.5-mm suture anchors, which are inserted into the posterior aspect of the calcaneus at the insertion of the Achilles tendon: 1 medial and 1 lateral (**Fig. 16**A, B). Although there are many suture options,

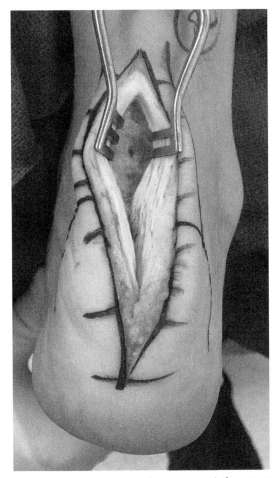

Fig. 9. A midline split in the tendon has been created for exposure and planned debridement.

it is the senior author's preference to use anchors each having 2 strands of #0 braided nonabsorbable Fiberwire (Arthrex, Naples, Florida) suture. Suture reaction has not been an issue with insertional Achilles procedures in the senior author's experience. These sutures are then used to reattach the Achilles tendon back down into the insertional region optimizing tendon to bone contact area (**Fig. 17**). The longitudinal split within the distal Achilles is then repaired using a #0 Fiberwire suture in a running fashion (**Fig. 18**). The paratenon is repaired as its own separate layer with #0 absorbable suture, and the skin is closed in layers.

    A sterile dressing is applied with the foot held in 20° of plantarflexion, and a padded posterior splint is applied to the leg.

PROGNOSTIC FACTORS

Some studies have shown that patients aged greater than 50 or 55 years have greater disease severity and inferior outcomes.[24,48] However, other studies have failed to show this association.[28,29] Additionally diabetics and obese patients have higher risks of wound complications following this procedure.[49,50]

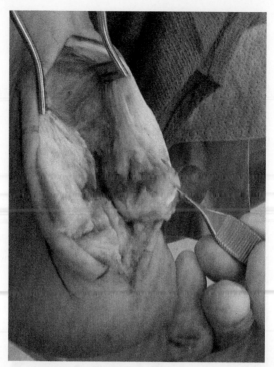

Fig. 10. Intraoperative photograph demonstrating thickening and calcification within the insertion of the Achilles tendon. The tendon has been split longitudinally and partially elevated off the insertion. The ventral surface appears tendinotic.

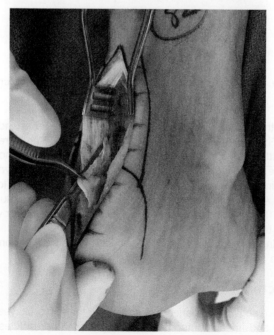

Fig. 11. The tendinotic portion of the Achilles tendon is debrided sharply to expose healthy tendon.

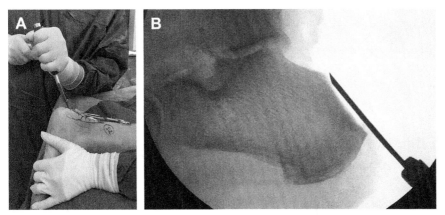

Fig. 12. An osteotome is used to resect the Haglund exostosis (A). Intraoperative fluoroscopy is used to demonstrate that a sufficient portion of bone is resected to avoid any further impingement on the Achilles tendon (B). The resection starts distal to the insertional spur, and care is taken to avoid violating the posterior facet of the subtalar joint.

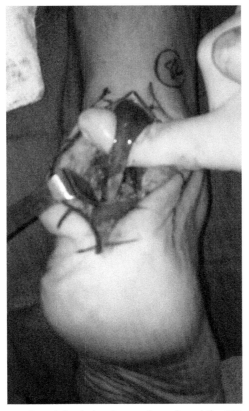

Fig. 13. The deep compartment fascia has been released, and the FHL tendon is identified.

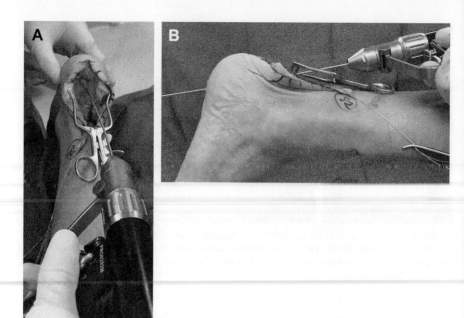

Fig. 14. A guide pin is passed from dorsal to plantar just anterior to the Achilles tendon insertion and marks the planned location for the FHL tendon transfer (*A, B*).

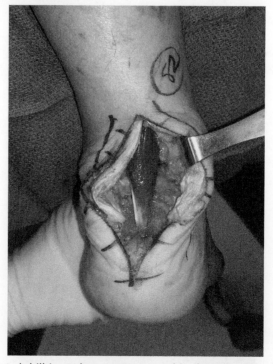

Fig. 15. A cannulated drill is used to create a tunnel in the calcaneal tuberosity over the guide pin, and then the FHL tendon is passed through the tunnel and secured with an interference screw.

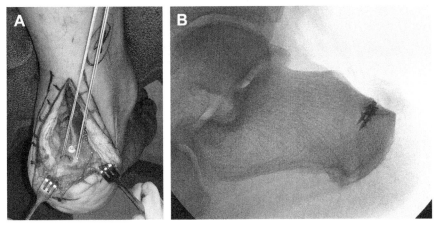

Fig. 16. Two suture anchors are placed in the calcaneal tuberosity (*A*), and intraoperative fluoroscopy confirms an appropriate position (*B*).

POSTOPERATIVE REHABILITATION

Early mobilization and weight-bearing is the trend after Achilles debridement and repair to minimize atrophy and allow for earlier return to activities, especially with improved methods for tendon fixation. A sample protocol after a central-splitting

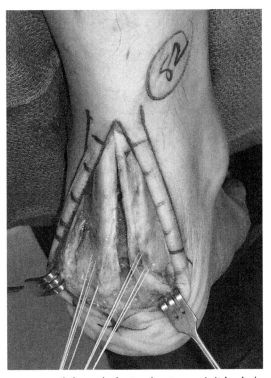

Fig. 17. The sutures are passed through the tendon to repair it back down to its insertion.

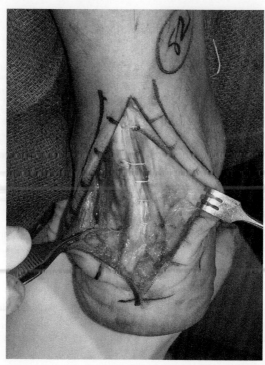

Fig. 18. A running permanent suture is then placed to repair the longitudinal split in the tendon.

approach with 2-anchor tendon repair includes 2 weeks of nonweight-bearing and splint immobilization followed by weight-bearing as tolerated in a boot with a heel wedge or a plantarflexion cast.[28] Patients are transitioned into a sneaker with a heel lift at 6 weeks postoperatively and initiate gastroc-soleus strengthening at 12 weeks without formal physical therapy. Transition out of the boot can be performed as early as 4 weeks postoperatively if the tendon is not fully detached from its insertion.[25] Full return to sports is variable, but usually requires a recovery time of 5 to 6 months.[26]

COMPLICATIONS

There is a 4.7% complication rate after surgery for insertional Achilles tendinopathy.[51] Wound healing issues tend to be the most common complications seen after surgery for insertional Achilles tendinopathy, reported in 3% to 31% of cases.[27,28,30,43] Most cases are managed nonsurgically with local wound care and oral antibiotics. FHL transfer may be associated with increased wound complications postoperatively.[30] Deep venous thrombosis (DVT) is thought to occur in a higher rate in Achilles procedures compared with other foot and ankle procedures. Nonetheless, the overall DVT rate reported is still low, ranging from 0% to 5%.[27,30,43] Hypertrophic or hypersensitivity along the scar may occur in up to 10% of cases.[26,43] Patients rarely need to return to the operating room because of a postoperative complication. Out of 138 patients in several published case series, 3 patients (2%) were taken back to the operating room postoperatively for irrigation and debridement of hematoma, mechanical failure of suture anchors and tendon repair, and repeat tendon debridement at 8 months respectively.[26–28,43]

SUMMARY

There are a variety of successful ways to surgically manage insertional Achilles tendinopathy. Thorough debridement is important in resolving patient symptoms, and this often requires near-complete detachment of the tendon. Repair using at least 2 suture anchors seems to be associated with optimal outcomes, and there is a theoretic and biomechanical benefit to using a double-row repair technique. The addition of an FHL transfer is not proven to be beneficial in the older population and may be associated with increased wound healing problems. With robust tendon repair following debridement, early weight-bearing and mobilization can be employed, allowing for earlier return to function. Return to sports is still typically delayed until 5 or 6 months postoperatively. Complications are rare, but when seen, are typically related to wound healing issues and superficial infections that do not require return to the operating room. Tendon debridement and repair are a successful procedure associated with high functional outcome scores in patients with recalcitrant insertional Achilles tendinopathy. Additional study is needed to determine the optimal components of the surgical treatment and whether expedited return to sports is possible with improved repair techniques.

REFERENCES

1. Clement DB, Taunton JE, Smart GW. Achilles tendinitis and peritendinitis: etiology and treatment. Am J Sports Med 1984;12(3):179–84.
2. Kvist M. Achilles tendon injuries in athletes. Ann Chir Gynaecol 1991;80(2): 188–201.
3. Holmes GB, Lin J. Etiologic factors associated with symptomatic achilles tendinopathy. Foot Ankle Int 2006;27(11):952–9.
4. Irwin TA. Current concepts review: insertional Achilles tendinopathy. Foot Ankle Int 2010;31(10):933–9.
5. Zanetti M, Metzdorf A, Kundert HP, et al. Achilles tendons: clinical relevance of neovascularization diagnosed with power Doppler US. Radiology 2003;227(2): 556–60.
6. Knobloch K, Kraemer R, Lichtenberg A, et al. Achilles tendon and paratendon microcirculation in midportion and insertional tendinopathy in athletes. Am J Sports Med 2006;34(1):92–7.
7. Rufai A, Ralphs JR, Benjamin M. Structure and histopathology of the insertional region of the human Achilles tendon. J Orthop Res 1995;13(4):585–93.
8. Schubert TE, Weidler C, Lerch K, et al. Achilles tendinosis is associated with sprouting of substance P positive nerve fibres. Ann Rheum Dis 2005;64(7): 1083–6.
9. Scott A, Lian O, Bahr R, et al. Increased mast cell numbers in human patellar tendinosis: correlation with symptom duration and vascular hyperplasia. Br J Sports Med 2008;42(9):753–7.
10. Kragsnaes MS, Fredberg U, Stribolt K, et al. Stereological quantification of immune-competent cells in baseline biopsy specimens from Achilles tendons: results from patients with chronic tendinopathy followed for more than 4 years. Am J Sports Med 2014;42(10):2435–45.
11. Lyman J, Weinhold PS, Almekinders LC. Strain behavior of the distal Achilles tendon: implications for insertional Achilles tendinopathy. Am J Sports Med 2004;32(2):457–61.
12. Kang S, Thordarson DB, Charlton TP. Insertional Achilles tendinitis and Haglund's deformity. Foot Ankle Int 2012;33(6):487–91.

13. Nicholson CW, Berlet GC, Lee TH. Prediction of the success of nonoperative treatment of insertional Achilles tendinosis based on MRI. Foot Ankle Int 2007; 28(4):472–7.

14. Lu CC, Cheng YM, Fu YC, et al. Angle analysis of Haglund syndrome and its relationship with osseous variations and Achilles tendon calcification. Foot Ankle Int 2007;28(2):181–5.

15. Benjamin M, Rufai A, Ralphs JR. The mechanism of formation of bony spurs (enthesophytes) in the Achilles tendon. Arthritis Rheum 2000;43(3):576–83.

16. Fowler A, Philip JF. Abnormality of the calcaneus as a cause of painful heel. Br J Surg 1945;32:494–8.

17. Pavlov H, Heneghan MA, Hersh A, et al. The Haglund syndrome: initial and differential diagnosis. Radiology 1982;144(1):83–8.

18. Haims AH, Schweitzer ME, Patel RS, et al. MR imaging of the Achilles tendon: overlap of findings in symptomatic and asymptomatic individuals. Skeletal Radiol 2000;29(11):640–5.

19. Astrom M, Gentz CF, Nilsson P, et al. Imaging in chronic Achilles tendinopathy: a comparison of ultrasonography, magnetic resonance imaging and surgical findings in 27 histologically verified cases. Skeletal Radiol 1996;25(7):615–20.

20. Fahlstrom M, Jonsson P, Lorentzon R, et al. Chronic Achilles tendon pain treated with eccentric calf-muscle training. Knee Surg Sports Traumatol Arthrosc 2003; 11(5):327–33.

21. Jonsson P, Alfredson H, Sunding K, et al. New regimen for eccentric calf-muscle training in patients with chronic insertional Achilles tendinopathy: results of a pilot study. Br J Sports Med 2008;42(9):746–9.

22. Rompe JD, Furia J, Maffulli N. Eccentric loading compared with shock wave treatment for chronic insertional Achilles tendinopathy. A randomized, controlled trial. J Bone Joint Surg Am 2008;90(1):52–61.

23. Yodlowski ML, Scheller AD Jr, Minos L. Surgical treatment of Achilles tendinitis by decompression of the retrocalcaneal bursa and the superior calcaneal tuberosity. Am J Sports Med 2002;30(3):318–21.

24. Watson AD, Anderson RB, Davis WH. Comparison of results of retrocalcaneal decompression for retrocalcaneal bursitis and insertional achilles tendinosis with calcific spur. Foot Ankle Int 2000;21(8):638–42.

25. Wagner E, Gould JS, Kneidel M, et al. Technique and results of Achilles tendon detachment and reconstruction for insertional Achilles tendinosis. Foot Ankle Int 2006;27(9):677–84.

26. Maffulli N, Testa V, Capasso G, et al. Calcific insertional Achilles tendinopathy: re-attachment with bone anchors. Am J Sports Med 2004;32(1):174–82.

27. Ettinger S, Razzaq R, Waizy H, et al. Operative treatment of the insertional Achilles tendinopathy through a transtendinous approach. Foot Ankle Int 2016;37(3): 288–93.

28. Nunley JA, Ruskin G, Horst F. Long-term clinical outcomes following the central incision technique for insertional Achilles tendinopathy. Foot Ankle Int 2011; 32(9):850–5.

29. Johnson KW, Zalavras C, Thordarson DB. Surgical management of insertional calcific Achilles tendinosis with a central tendon splitting approach. Foot Ankle Int 2006;27(4):245–50.

30. Hunt KJ, Cohen BE, Davis WH, et al. Surgical treatment of insertional Achilles tendinopathy with or without flexor hallucis longus tendon transfer: a prospective, randomized study. Foot Ankle Int 2015;36(9):998–1005.

31. Beitzel K, Mazzocca AD, Obopilwe E, et al. Biomechanical properties of double- and single-row suture anchor repair for surgical treatment of insertional Achilles tendinopathy. Am J Sports Med 2013;41(7):1642–8.

32. Pilson H, Brown P, Stitzel J, et al. Single-row versus double-row repair of the distal Achilles tendon: a biomechanical comparison. J Foot Ankle Surg 2012;51(6): 762–6.

33. Fanter NJ, Davis EW, Baker CL Jr. Fixation of the Achilles tendon insertion using suture button technology. Am J Sports Med 2012;40(9):2085–91.

34. Cox JT, Shorten PL, Gould GC, et al. Knotted versus knotless suture bridge repair of the achilles tendon insertion: a biomechanical study. Am J Sports Med 2014; 42(11):2727–33.

35. Finni T, Komi PV, Lukkariniemi J. Achilles tendon loading during walking: application of a novel optic fiber technique. Eur J Appl Physiol Occup Physiol 1998; 77(3):289–91.

36. Wapner KL, Pavlock GS, Hecht PJ, et al. Repair of chronic Achilles tendon rupture with flexor hallucis longus tendon transfer. Foot Ankle 1993;14(8):443–9.

37. Hahn F, Meyer P, Maiwald C, et al. Treatment of chronic Achilles tendinopathy and ruptures with flexor hallucis tendon transfer: clinical outcome and MRI findings. Foot Ankle Int 2008;29(8):794–802.

38. Martin RL, Manning CM, Carcia CR, et al. An outcome study of chronic Achilles tendinosis after excision of the Achilles tendon and flexor hallucis longus tendon transfer. Foot Ankle Int 2005;26(9):691–7.

39. Wilcox DK, Bohay DR, Anderson JG. Treatment of chronic achilles tendon disorders with flexor hallucis longus tendon transfer/augmentation. Foot Ankle Int 2000;21(12):1004–10.

40. Kolodziej P, Glisson RR, Nunley JA. Risk of avulsion of the Achilles tendon after partial excision for treatment of insertional tendonitis and Haglund's deformity: a biomechanical study. Foot Ankle Int 1999;20(7):433–7.

41. Den Hartog BD. Flexor hallucis longus transfer for chronic Achilles tendonosis. Foot Ankle Int 2003;24(3):233–7.

42. Elias I, Raikin SM, Besser MP, et al. Outcomes of chronic insertional Achilles tendinosis using FHL autograft through single incision. Foot Ankle Int 2009;30(3): 197–204.

43. Schon LC, Shores JL, Faro FD, et al. Flexor hallucis longus tendon transfer in treatment of Achilles tendinosis. J Bone Joint Surg Am 2013;95(1):54–60.

44. Hansen S. Trauma to the heel cord. In: Jahss M, editor. Disorders of the foot and ankle. 2nd edition. Philadelphia: WB Saunders; 1991. p. 2355–60.

45. Will RE, Galey SM. Outcome of single incision flexor hallucis longus transfer for chronic Achilles tendinopathy. Foot Ankle Int 2009;30(4):315–7.

46. Georgiannos D, Lampridis V, Vasiliadis A, et al. Treatment of insertional Achilles pathology with dorsal wedge calcaneal osteotomy in athletes. Foot Ankle Int 2017;38(4):381–7.

47. Zadek I. An operation for the cure of achillobursitis. Am J Surg 1939;43(2):542–6.

48. McGarvey WC, Palumbo RC, Baxter DE, et al. Insertional Achilles tendinosis: surgical treatment through a central tendon splitting approach. Foot Ankle Int 2002; 23(1):19–25.

49. Saxena A, Maffulli N, Nguyen A, et al. Wound complications from surgeries pertaining to the Achilles tendon: an analysis of 219 surgeries. J Am Podiatr Med Assoc 2008;98(2):95–101.

50. Burrus MT, Werner BC, Yarboro SR. Obesity is associated with increased postoperative complications after operative management of tibial shaft fractures. Injury 2016;47(2):465–70.

51. Paavola M, Orava S, Leppilahti J, et al. Chronic Achilles tendon overuse injury: complications after surgical treatment. An analysis of 432 consecutive patients. Am J Sports Med 2000;28(1):77–82.

Using Arthroscopic Techniques for Achilles Pathology

Rebecca Cerrato, MD[a], Paul Switaj, MD[b]

KEYWORDS

- Arthroscopic • Achilles • Chronic Achilles rupture • Tendinopathy

KEY POINTS

- Endoscopically assisted procedures have been established to provide the surgeon with minimally invasive techniques to address common Achilles conditions.
- Modifications to some of these techniques as well as improvements in instrumentation have allowed these procedures to provide similar clinical results to the traditional open surgeries while reducing wound complications and accelerating patient's recoveries.
- The available literature on these techniques reports consistently good outcomes with few complications, making them appealing for surgeons to adopt.

INTRODUCTION

Endoscopic procedures around the foot and ankle provide the surgeon with the techniques to treat a variety of pathology with a minimally invasive approach. These less-invasive approaches can diminish scar tissue and result in less perioperative pain, fewer wound complications, and quicker recovery.

Special focus has been placed on the Achilles tendon complex, where these techniques have been used to address acute and chronic ruptures, equinus contractures, and both insertional and noninsertional tendinopathies. Although high-level evidence-based literature for Achilles tendoscopy is somewhat lacking, the literature available does report consistently good outcomes with few complications, making them appealing for surgeons to adopt.

ANATOMY

Knowledge of the local anatomy is mandatory for reducing complications when surgically addressing pathology of the Achilles tendon. The Achilles tendon is the longest

Dr R. Cerrato Paid consultant for Wright Medical Technology, Depuy Synthes. Dr P. Switaj Nothing to disclose.
[a] Mercy Medical Center, The Institute for Foot and Ankle Reconstruction, 301 St. Paul Place, Baltimore, MD 21202, USA; [b] Orthovirginia, 1850 Town Center Parkway, Suite 400, Reston, VA 20190, USA
E-mail address: rcerrato@mdmercy.com

and most powerful tendon in the human body, measuring 12 cm to 15 cm in length and up to 2.5 cm in diameter.[1] It is the confluence of the soleus and gastrocnemius muscle aponeuroses, and, rarely, the plantaris.[2] These muscles are both innervated by the tibial nerve, and together form the gastrocnemius-soleus complex, or triceps surae.

The soleus lies deep to the gastrocnemius and superficial to the muscles of the deep posterior compartment. The gastrocnemius muscle originates off the distal femur and crosses the knee, ankle, and subtalar joint before inserting broadly onto the calcaneus approximately 13 mm inferior to the most proximal margin of the tuberosity.[3] Thus, when the knee is extended, the gastrocnemius limits dorsiflexion, whereas when the knee is flexed, the entire triceps surae can limit dorsiflexion. Prior investigators have divided the surgical anatomy into 5 levels. Level 5 consists of proximal insertions of the gastrocnemius. Level 4 comprises the muscle bellies of the gastrocnemius. Level 3 begins where the muscle bellies of the gastrocnemius coalesce and finishes where the aponeuroses of the soleus and gastrocnemius combine. Level 2 starts in the common aponeurotic tendon of the soleus and gastrocnemius and finishes at the distal end of the soleus muscle. Level 1 consists of the Achilles tendon.[2,4]

As the tendon courses distally, the fibers rotate, giving it greater mechanical resistance, but creating a poorly vascularized area 2 to 6 cm proximal to its insertion.[5,6] The posterior tibial artery is the major blood supply to the proximal and distal sections of the tendon, whereas the peroneal artery has fewer vessels and supplies the midsection.[7] This vascular anatomy may predispose the Achilles to degeneration in this area. In addition, the Achilles tendon does not have a true tendon sheath, but is surrounded by paratenon. This paratenon is separated into 3 layers: the inner visceral, the mesotendon, and outer parietal layers. The retrocalcaneal bursa allows for proper gliding of the Achilles tendon and lies between the tendon and the calcaneus at its insertion point. Both the paratenon and the retrocalcaneal bursa can be sites of ongoing inflammation that can cause substantial morbidity to patients.

BIOMECHANICS

Contraction of the gastrocnemius-soleus complex produces plantarflexion of the ankle combined with adduction and internal rotation of the foot.[2] The flexion force of the gastrocnemius is greater when the knee joint is fully extended, because it crosses the knee joint. The soleus delivers more than twice the plantarflexion force of the gastrocnemius, whose medial head provides most of its power, with the lateral head only accounting for 29% of the power.[8] Overall, the Achilles tendon sustains up to 12.5 times of body weight during certain running activities.[3]

ACUTE PATHOLOGY
Achilles Rupture

Ruptures of the Achilles tendon represent one of the most common sport injuries. Although a thorough discussion of the surgical versus nonsurgical treatment is beyond the scope of this review article, investigators have cited increased wound complications,[9] significant risk of infection, and scar formation at the site of repair.[10] Because of these risks, other minimally invasive approaches have been developed. Ma and Griffith[9] first introduced this idea in 1977, which has been modified throughout the years.[11,12] Unfortunately, some of the earlier reports on these techniques had reported a higher complication rate, including increased rate of rerupture and increased sural nerve injuries.[13] These earlier percutaneous techniques also do not allow for visual evaluation of the repair site or tendon quality, which may result in poor approximation of the tendon ends. Newer technology allows the surgeon to view the repair and place a jig within the paratenon, allowing suture passage without capturing the sural nerve.[11] To address earlier concerns with the percutaneous techniques, endoscopic-assisted methods have been introduced. These methods allow the surgeon to evaluate the tendon quality, adequate mobilize the stumps, ensure accurate needle passage, and confirm approximation of the tendon ends.

Technique
The patient is placed in a prone position, and a pneumatic thigh tourniquet is placed. The resting plantarflexion of contralateral extremity is examined with the knee flexed. In the author's experience, they tension their acute Achilles ruptures in maximum plantarflexion and have not experienced any instances of "overtightening." The rupture gap is outlined. Halasi and colleagues[14] described a modified Ma-Griffith technique, with 6 skin incisions, 2 scope portals, and a double suture construct (**Fig. 1**). The technique uses no. 2 Vicryl (other investigators have described variations to this repair using nonabsorbable suture, such as EthiBond). Six incisions are marked, 2 above the rupture both medial and lateral at the proximal stump, 2 at the rupture gap, and 2 below the rupture both medial and lateral at the distal stump. The 2 incisions at the tendon gap can be used for the endoscopic portals. The suture is passed using

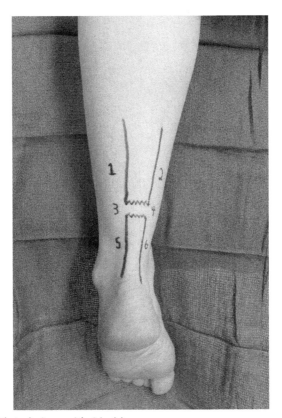

Fig. 1. Ma-Griffith technique with 6 incisions.

a straight needle. To protect the sural nerve, the investigators used a small drill sleeve as a soft tissue protector. The soft tissue protector is placed directly on the paratenon through the skin incisions. The same 6 incisions can be used to place both suture strands (**Fig. 2**). The endoscopic portals are created at the 2 central incisions directly at the rupture gap. A 4.0-mm 30° or 2.7-mm 30° scope is introduced first laterally, and the second portal incision is created at the gap. The tear is inspected; hematoma is evacuated, and if necessary, the tendon ends debrided. The surgery should be performed with low-pressure gravity inflow to prevent excessive fluid extravasation and compartment syndrome. Tendon end reapproximation can be visualized with suture tensioning. Once the double suture construct is completed, the ankle is held in plantarflexion and the sutures tied.

Postoperative care

Postoperative protocol included 3 weeks of non-weight-bearing in an equinus short leg cast, followed by weight-bearing in a walking brace with a lifted heel for an additional 5 weeks and functional rehabilitation initiated as well.[14]

CLINICAL RESULTS

Turgut and colleagues[15] first reported endoscopic-assisted techniques in 2002. Since then, other studies have demonstrated satisfactory results with differing suture

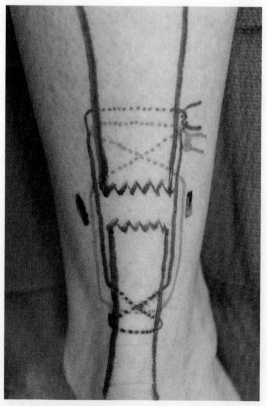

Fig. 2. Percutaneous Achilles rupture repair. Halasi modification with double suture construct included the *3* and *4* marked incisions as the location for the endoscopic portals.

techniques.[10,12,14–19] There has been one level II study by Halasi and colleagues[14] comparing a group of patients undergoing percutaneous Achilles repair with the use of endoscopy to a group undergoing the same procedure without endoscopy. Both groups yielded similar clinical results, including comparable strength, calf atrophy, and return to activities. The endoscopy group had lower, but nonsignificant, rate of rerupture (1.75% vs 5.7%), which the group attributed to improved visualization and control of the tendons ends (**Table 1**).

CHRONIC PATHOLOGY
Equinus Contracture

Contracture of the gastrocnemius-soleus complex has been associated with a multitude of foot and ankle pathologies, both as the root cause and in conjunction with other deformities.[20,21] An equinus contracture is a limitation in ankle dorsiflexion not caused by bony ankle pathology. It may be secondary to a global contracture of the gastrocnemius-soleus complex or isolated to the gastrocnemius muscle alone. Because the gastrocnemius crosses the knee joint, the contributions of both units can be differentiated on physical examination with the Silfverskiold test. The test is considered positive when, with the subtalar joint held in a neutral position, there is limited dorsiflexion with the knee extended that improves with the knee flexed. The most commonly used criterion to indicate an isolated gastrocnemius contracture is less than 10° of dorsiflexion with the knee extended, which improves with knee flexion.[20]

Isolated contractures of the gastrocnemius have long been treated by open techniques, whereas the tendo-Achilles lengthening is often addressed in a percutaneous manner. These techniques sometimes led to delayed wound healing, sural nerve irritation, undesirable scar formation, and tethering of the skin to the crural fascia. The described endoscopic techniques are focused on addressing the gastrocnemius contracture.

Technique

Endoscopic gastrocnemius recession was first described in a cadaveric model in 2003 by Tashjian and colleagues.[22]

The patient is placed either prone or supine on the operating room table with a thigh tourniquet. The position is most often dictated by other concomitant procedures being performed.

Endoscopy, which can be performed using 1 or 2 entry points, should ensure that the cannula is placed between the sural fascia and the aponeuroses of the insertion of the gastrocnemius to enable recession of the fascia. An alternative technique has been described in which the intramuscular portion of the aponeuroses is released instead.[23]

Medial portal placement has been anatomically detailed in many articles and is performed at the anatomic level 3, where the muscle bellies of the gastrocnemius coalesce. This placement is crucial to a successful, complication-free operation and has been described as 2 cm distal to the indent of the musculotendinous junction,[22,24] 16 to 17 cm proximal to the distal tip of the medial malleolus,[25] just distal to the junction of the middle and distal thirds of the leg,[26] and 4 fingerbreadths proximal to the flare of the medial malleolus.[27]

The medial portal is established, and a curved hemostat is used to puncture the cural fascia overlying the superficial posterior compartment. The blunt trocar with a slotted cannula is introduced and advanced laterally. The lateral portal is established in an inside-out technique. The trochar is removed, leaving the slotted

Table 1
Clinical studies on endoscopic Achilles rupture repair

Author, Year	No. of Procedures	Clinical Outcomes	Complications	Comments
Turgut et al,[15] 2002	11	100% satisfactory results	No reruptures, wound issues, or nerve injury	
Halasi et al,[14] 2003	57	89% good-excellent	1 partial rerupture; 4 fusiform thickening; 1 DVT	Mean plantarflexion strength 86% of contralateral side
Tang et al,[16] 2007	20	75% excellent, 25% good according to Arner-Lindholm scale	No reruptures, wound issues, or nerve injury	Follow-up MRI demonstrated good repair of all tendons
Fortis et al,[10] 2008	20	100% good-excellent; mean postoperative Merkel score 604	10% sural neuralgic; 1 subsided with no further treatment	
Doral et al,[17] 2009	62	94% excellent, 6% good; mean postoperative AOFAS score 94.6	3.2% sural nerve hypoesthesia, all resolved spontaneously	95% return to prior sporting activities
Chiu et al,[18] 2013	19	94.8% excellent results	1 superficial infection, 2 sural nerve hypoesthesia	95% return to prior sporting activities

Abbreviation: DVT, deep vein thrombosis.

cannula. A 4.0-mm 30° arthroscope is inserted medially and the gastrocnemius aponeurosis is inspected. The lens is rotated 180°, and the sural nerve and lesser saphenous veins are visualized. It is important to identify that the sural nerve is posterior to the cannula; otherwise, it can be inadvertently cut. The ankle is held in maximum dorsiflexion to tension the Achilles. A retrograde hook blade is introduced into the slotted cannula laterally. The gastrocnemius aponeurosis is released from medial to lateral. The ankle is passively dorsiflexed to confirm adequate release.

Postoperative care

Isolated gastrocnemius recessions can be allowed weight-bearing immediately in a walking boot, although some investigators describe a 2-week period in a non-weight-bearing splint. A 90° night splint is prescribed, and ankle dorsiflexion exercises are encouraged. Typically, patients are weaned out of the boot at 4 weeks, and physical therapy is initiated. For patients with concomitant procedures, splinting and weight-bearing restrictions were directed by those.

CLINICAL RESULTS

Overall, good outcomes have been described using both 1- and 2-portal techniques. The first clinical series was described in 2004 by Saxena and Widtfeldt[28] and demonstrated a mean increase in dorsiflexion of 12.6°, but with 3 out of 18 patients experiencing sural dysesthesias. All except one of the patients underwent associated procedures at the time of gastrocnemius recession. Subsequent series have consistently demonstrated significant increases in dorsiflexion as well as improved outcome measures.[25–27,29–34] The largest series to date from Phisitkul and colleagues[33] demonstrated mean ankle dorsiflexion improvement from $-0.8 \pm 5.4°$ preoperatively to $11.0 \pm 6.6°$ at an average of 13 months postoperatively. Postoperative weakness in plantarflexion and sural nerve dysesthesias occurred in 3.1% and 3.4%, respectively, without any wound complications or Achilles tendon rupture (**Table 2**).

One study performed in 23 diabetic patients using a uniportal technique showed 3 conversions to open procedures, 3 delayed wound healing, and 3 undercorrections (although this was not objectively defined) without any nerve injuries.[35] The most recent study by Thevendran and colleagues[34] on 54 feet demonstrated 3 cases of unsatisfactory scar, 3 cases of sural nerve dysesthesia, and 3 cases of subjective plantar flexion weakness, while Schroeder[32] showed a 1.67% incidence of persistence sural nerve injury and no wound healing or scar problems. Phisitkul and colleagues[33] reported the largest series to date, noting a 3.1% incidence of weakness of ankle plantarflexion and 3.4% incidence of sural nerve dysesthesia without any wound complications in 320 patients.

Endoscopy provides a better cosmetic outcome, although it carries a considerable risk of sural nerve injury. The complication rate can reach 22.2%. The importance of the association between the sural nerve and the endoscopic entry point led to the study by Tashjian and colleagues,[22] who found the distance between the sural nerve and the lateral border of the gastrocnemius and soleus to be 12 mm (range, 7–17 mm). This short distance justifies the use of a medial entry point in this type of endoscopic procedure.

Noninsertional Achilles Tendinopathy

Noninsertional Achilles disorders typically occur 4 cm to 6 cm proximal to its insertion and comprise midportion tendinosis as well as acute and chronic paratendinopathy. It is important to correctly diagnosis peritendinitis. On physical examination, the pain

Table 2
Clinical studies on endoscopic gastrocnemius recession

Author, Year	No. of Procedures	Range of Motion (Degrees)/ Clinical Outcomes	Complications	Comments
Saxena & Widtfeldt,[28] 2004	18	−8.7° → 3.6°	3 sural dysesthesias	Only one isolated recession
DiDomenico et al,[29] 2005	31	Mean increase 18°		
Trevino et al,[26] 2005	28	Modified O&M scores statistically significant improvement (8 patients able to be contacted)	1 superficial wound infection, 1 conversion to open	2 incorrect locations of portal placement necessitating second incision
Saxena et al,[30] 2007	54	−8° → 7°	1 hematoma, 1 overlengthening, 6 skin tenting, 6 lateral foot dysesthesias	Most patients with additional reconstructive procedures
Grady & Kelly,[31] 2010	40	Mean increase 15°	No sural nerve complications	Patients 18 y old and younger
Roukis & Schweinberger,[35] 2010	23		3 delayed healing, 3 undercorrections, 3 conversions to open	Focused only on complications; patient all had diabetes
Yeap et al,[27] 2011				
Angthong & Kanitnate,[25] 2012	4	Mean increase 35°/significant improvements in AOFAS, VAS-FA scores	None	Severe equinus deformities in 3 patients combined with percutaneous TAL
Schroeder,[32] 2012	60	−2.9° → 12.8°	3 nerve complications (2 resolved), 1 weakness	
Phisitkul et al,[33] 2014	344	−0.8° → 11.0°/significant improvements in VAS, SF-36, and FFI	3.2% weakness of plantarflexion, 3.4% sural dysesthesias	No difference between isolated and combined procedures
Lui,[23] 2015				Technique paper
Thevendran et al,[34] 2015	56	Significant improvements in SF-36, AOFAS hindfoot, modified O&M, and VAS, 91% good or very good outcomes	3 unsatisfactory scar, 3 sural dysesthesias, 5 subjective plantar flexion weakness	

Abbreviations: FFI, foot function index; O&M, Olerud and Molander; SF-36, Short Form 36; VAS, visual analogue score–foot and ankle.

remains in a specific location during ankle dorsiflexion and plantarflexion with peritendinitis, while the pain moves with the tendon in tendinosis.

Initial conservative treatment incorporating an eccentric therapy program is often successful, but can still fail to provide adequate symptom relief in almost one-third of patients.[36] A variety of surgical procedures have been described, including open debridement with or without stripping of the paratenon, percutaneous longitudinal tenotomy, plantaris release, and isolated gastrocnemius recession. These open approaches have been associated with wound complications, prolonged recovery, and scarring.[37] Thus, endoscopic techniques have been developed to achieve the goals of open surgery, excising areas of degeneration, adhesions, and thickened paratenon, and stimulating a healing response, while decreasing the morbidity.

Technique
The patient is positioned prone on the operating table with a thigh tourniquet. Their feet are positioned off the table, allowing ankle dorsiflexion and plantarflexion during the procedure.

The borders of the Achilles tendon and the superior aspect of the calcaneal tuberosity are marked out with a surgical pen. Several variations in portal placement have been described.[38,39] Typically, 2 portals are used. Maquirriain[38] described using a proximal portal 10 cm above the Achilles insertion of the calcaneus at the midline of the Achilles. The distal portal is placed again midline, at the distal location, not to disrupt the confluence of the Achilles and the skin as it nears attachment. Thermann and colleagues[39] described placing portals at the medial edge of the Achilles. Other have described a similar 2-portal technique placed lateral to the Achilles border, placed approximately 2 to 4 cm proximal and distal to the pathologic thickening on the Achilles.

A 4.0- or 2.7-mm 30° arthroscope is introduced into the proximal portal, and a dry tendon inspection is performed. Gravity inflow is then used for insufflation. The distal portal is established with the aid of direct visualization using the scope. In cases of peritendinitis, the peritendon is released, paying particular attention to releasing the anterior aspect of the tendon. In cases with tendinosis, following debridement, longitudinal incisions are made in the diseased segment of the tendon using a retrograde blade.

Postoperative care
For patients with a peritendon release and debridement only, most investigators allow immediate weight-bearing in a walker boot. Active ankle dorsiflexion and plantarflexion are encouraged. Eccentric stretching exercises are initiated after 2 weeks. For patients that underwent tenotomies, they are placed in a walker boot and kept non-weight-bearing for up to 2 weeks.

CLINICAL RESULTS

Maquirriain[38] first described the use of endoscopic treatment of chronic Achilles tendinopathy in 1998 in a cadaveric model. Maquirriain followed his cadaveric research with a small clinic series demonstrating satisfactory results.[40] Additional investigators have published small series with satisfactory results and no reported complications.[15,39,41–44] Maquirriain[45] more recently reviewed his results on 27 patients, reporting improved outcomes and 2 complications (**Table 3**).

Insertional Achilles Tendinopathy

These disorders include pathology within the first 2 cm proximal to the insertion to the calcaneus. Although these disorders include insertional Achilles tendinosis and superficial calcaneal bursitis, endoscopic treatment has focused on treating retrocalcaneal

Table 3
Clinical studies on endoscopic chronic Achilles pathology

Author, Year	No. of Procedures	Pathology	Outcomes	Comments
Maquirriain et al,[40] 2002	7	2 peritendinitis, 4 midportion tendinosis, 1 chronic partial tear	Improvement in Achilles score from mean 39 to mean 89	1 minor hematoma with spontaneous resolution. Postoperative MRI in tendinosis patient with improvement
Morag et al,[41] 2003	4	2 posttraumatic adhesions, 2 midportion tendinosis	4–6 wk return to daily activities, 4 mo return to sporting activity	No complications
Vega et al,[42] 2008	8	Midportion tendinosis without rupture	All patients pain-free at last follow-up, 100% excellent results with Nelen scale	No complications; all patients returned to prior sporting activities
Thermann et al,[39] 2009	8	Midportion tendinosis	Pain improved from 40 to 97.5, Achilles function from 22.5 to 90	No complications
Liu,[43] 2012	20	Midportion tendinosis	ATSS-17 improved from 29.4 to 89	No complications
Pearce et al,[44] 2012	11	Mid-portion tendinosis	AOFAS improved from 68 to 92 postoperative, mean SF-36 scores also improved but were not statistically significant; 8/11 satisfied	No complications
Maquirriain,[45] 2013	27	Mid-portion tendinosis	VISA-A score improved from 37.0 to 97.5; the Achilles Tendon Scoring System score improved from 32.6 to 97.2	1 delayed keloid lesion, 1 seroma with chronic fistula

Abbreviations: ATTS-17, Achilles Tendinopathy Scoring System; VISA-A, Victorian Institute Sport Assessment-Achilles.

bursitis and associated Haglund deformity. Nonoperative treatment consists of physical therapy, shoe wear modifications, heel inserts, rest, anti-inflammatory drugs, and immobilization. However, there is a certain population of patients who fail to respond to nonsurgical measures.[46]

Open treatment traditionally includes open debridement of the tendon, retrocalcaneal bursectomy, and calcaneal exostectomy. Complications from these open procedures can include wound dehiscence, nerve irritation, and postoperative stiffness from extensive dissection. For patients with extensive insertional Achilles tendinopathy, these open approaches are preferred in order to perform an adequate debridement of the tendon, and reattachment if necessary.

Preoperative evaluation is vital to ensuring optimal, predictable results. In patients with isolated tenderness to palpation at the posterosuperior calcaneal border, and without significant intrasubstance changes on MRI evaluation, endoscopic calcaneoplasty may offer decreased wound-healing complications and the potential for quicker recovery time and decreased morbidity.

Technique

The patient can be placed either prone or supine on the operating room table with a thigh tourniquet. The positioning is the physician's preference. Regardless of patient position, appropriate setup is critical. The surgeon should make sure that there is enough space between the operative and contralateral extremity to ensure full freedom of motion with the arthroscope, without abutting the contralateral extremity. For prone positioning, the feet should be allowed to hang over the end of the surgical table and be elevated to allow medial portal instrument manipulation without crowding from the contralateral limb (**Fig. 3**). In supine positioning, the operative leg rests in a well-padded leg holder with the foot free floating. A surgical pen should be used to outline the Achilles and calcaneus.

Two portals, posteromedial and posterolateral, are commonly used with investigators describing additional accessory portals to aid in the visualization. The posterolateral porter is located typically 1 cm above the Achilles insertion and 0.5 cm below the superior aspect of the Haglund tubercle, adjacent to the tendon border (**Fig. 4**). A 5-mm vertical incision is made, and a hemostat is used to perform a spread-and-nick technique into the retrocalcaneal space. Either a 4-mm or a 2.7-mm 30° arthroscope

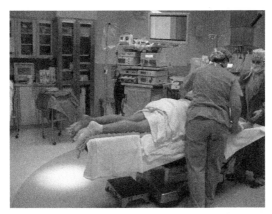

Fig. 3. Patient positioned prone for endoscopic Haglund with foot placed over operative table.

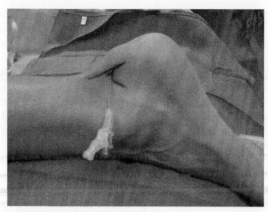

Fig. 4. Portal position for endoscopic Haglund.

is introduced. A gravity fluid system is used to avoid excessive soft tissue distention. A needle is placed through the marked posteromedial portal, at the same level as the posterolateral portal, and is visualized with the scope. An arthroscopic shaver is introduced, and the retrocalcaneal bursa, synovitis, and hyalinized tissue over the Haglund tubercle are debrided. Both portals are used interchangeably. An arthroscopic hooded or bone rasp is used to resect the tubercle to its insertion point on the calcaneus (**Figs. 5–8**). Some techniques have described this resection with visualization using the arthroscope, whereas others have performed the resection using flouroscopic guidance (**Fig. 9**). The diseased Achilles tissue can be debrided with the shaver.

Postoperative care
Patients can be splinted in equinus for the first 10 to 14 days, although several investigators discuss placing their patients in a walking boot with a 1-inch heel lift

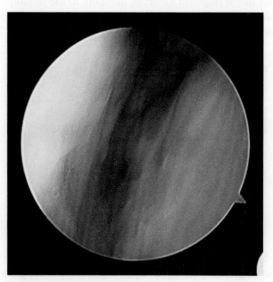

Fig. 5. Calcaneus covered with hyalinized tissue.

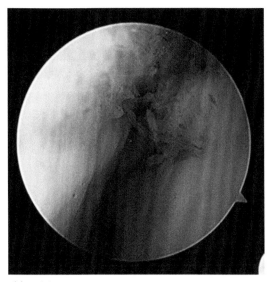

Fig. 6. Retrocalaneal bursitis.

immediately after surgery and permit weight-bearing as tolerated. Patients ambulate in the walking boot for 4 to 6 weeks and then transition to shoes with a heel lift.

CLINICAL RESULTS

Endoscopic calcaneoplasty was first described in 20 patients by van Dijk and colleagues[47] in 2001. Since then, multiple studies have been published demonstrating good success with endoscopic calcaneoplasty in patients with retrocalcaneal bursitis and a painful prominence of the posterosuperior aspect of the calcaneus.[48–55] Only a single level II study, by Leitze and colleagues,[49] has

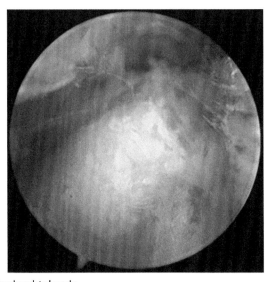

Fig. 7. Exposed Haglund tubercle.

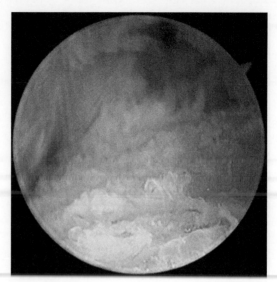

Fig. 8. Resected Haglund tubercle.

compared endoscopic with traditional open techniques. This study found that both compared experienced significant improvements in functional outcomes, without any significant differences between the groups in scores or time to recovery. The endoscopic procedures were associated with fewer complications than the open procedures (**Table 4**).

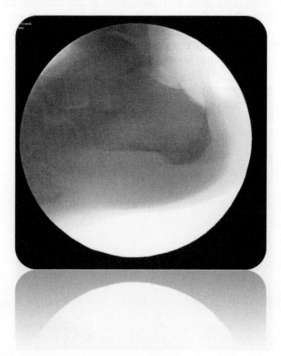

Fig. 9. Fluoroscopic assessment of Haglund resection.

Table 4
Clinical studies on endoscopic calcaneoplasty

Author, Year	No. of Procedures	Clinical Outcomes	Complications	Comments
van Dijk et al,[47] 2001	21	15 excellent, 4 good, 1 fair result	None	12 wk until return to sporting activities, 1 fair result in patient with cavovarus deformity
Jerosch & Nasef,[48] 2003	10	7 excellent, 4 good result in Ogilvie-Harris scores	None	No cavovarus deformity
Leitze et al,[49] 2003	33	Significant improvement in AOFAS-hindfoot; no significant differences in outcomes compared with open group with similar recovery time	3% infection (12% open), 10% altered sensation (18% open), 7% scar tenderness (18% open)	Compared with open technique
Jerosch et al,[50] 2007	81	41 excellent, 34 good, 3 fair results in Ogilvie-Harris scores	No neurovascular complications	No cavovarus deformity
Ortmann & McBryde,[51] 2007	32	AOFAS 62 → 97; 26 excellent, 3 good, 1 poor result	1 Achilles rupture 3 wk after surgery	1 residual pain requiring secondary open procedure
Jerosch et al,[52] 2012	164	84 excellent, 71 good, 5 patients fair, 4 poor results in Ogilvie-Harris score		
Kondreddi et al,[53] 2012	25	16 excellent, 6 good, 3 fair results; AOFAS 57 → 89		Patients with noninsertional tendinosis on ultrasound had worse results
Wu et al,[54] 2012	25	AOFAS 63 → 87; 15 excellent, 7 good, 1 fair, 2 poor results in Ogilvie-Harris score	None reported	
Kaynak et al,[55] 2013	30	AOFAS 53 → 99; all patients satisfied	None	

Chronic Achilles Rupture

Last, endoscopic techniques have been developed in order to address more complex issues with the Achilles tendon. Chronic Achilles ruptures can cause significant weakness in plantarflexion strength with resultant difficulty in walking inclines and poor balance.

Many methods to repair chronic Achilles ruptures have been described, including V-Y advancement, fascial turndown flaps, autologous tendon transfers, and allograft reconstructions. These techniques require large exposures with resultant problems with wound infection and nerve irritation,[56] especially in high-risk individuals such as diabetics, smokers, and those on disease-modifying medications for inflammatory arthropathy. In these patient populations, endoscopic techniques may have even greater benefit.

Gossage and colleagues[57] first described an endoscopic technique for a flexor hallucis longus (FHL) short harvest and transfer in the setting of 2 patients with chronic Achilles tendon ruptures, with good results and no complications. Lui and colleagues[58] published an endoscopic technique to perform a long harvest of the FHL tendon just proximal to the master knot of Henry, or down at the level of the proximal phalanx of the great toe.

Gedam and colleagues[59] used endoscopy to assist with a central turndown flap with semitendinosus augmentation in 14 patients with chronic ruptures with a mean gap of 5.1 cm. They showed American Orthopaedic Foot & Ankle Society (AOFAS) score improvement from 64.5 to 96.9 and Achilles Tendon Total Rupture Score improvement from 49.4 to 91.4, with no wound complications, nerve damage, or rerupture at a mean follow-up of 30.1 months. Piontek and colleagues[60] recently presented a technique of endoscopic Achilles reconstruction using autograft semitendinosus and gracilis tendons without any clinical results. They used a bone tunnel in the calcaneus and a tendon weave in the proximal stump in the Achilles tendon to achieve their tendon fixation.

SUMMARY

Endoscopically assisted procedures have been established to provide the surgeon with minimally invasive techniques to address common Achilles conditions. Modifications to some of these techniques as well as improvements in instrumentation have allowed these procedures to provide similar clinical results to the traditional open surgeries while reducing wound complications and accelerating patient's recoveries.

REFERENCES

1. Cummins EJ, Anson BJ. The structure of the calcaneal tendon (of Achilles) in relation to orthopedic surgery, with additional observations on the plantaris muscle. Surg Gynecol Obstet 1946;83:107–16.
2. Dalmau-Pastor M, Fargues-Polo B Jr, Casanova-Martinez D Jr, et al. Anatomy of the triceps surae: a pictorial essay. Foot Ankle Clin 2014;19:603–35.
3. Kelikian AS, Sarrafian SK, Sarrafian SK. Sarrafian's anatomy of the foot and ankle: descriptive, topographical, functional. 3rd edition. Philadelphia: Wolters Kluwer Health/Lippincott Williams & Wilkins; 2011.
4. Lamm BM, Paley D, Herzenberg JE. Gastrocnemius soleus recession: a simpler, more limited approach. J Am Podiatr Med Assoc 2005;95:18–25.
5. Doral MN, Alam M, Bozkurt M, et al. Functional anatomy of the Achilles tendon. Knee Surg Sports Traumatol Arthrosc 2010;18:638–43.

6. Lagergren C, Lindholm A. Vascular distribution in the Achilles tendon; an angiographic and microangiographic study. Acta Chir Scand 1959;116:491–5.
7. Chen TM, Rozen WM, Pan WR, et al. The arterial anatomy of the Achilles tendon: anatomical study and clinical implications. Clin Anat 2009;22:377–85.
8. Silver RL, de la Garza J, Rang M. The myth of muscle balance. A study of relative strengths and excursions of normal muscles about the foot and ankle. J Bone Joint Surg Br 1985;67:432–7.
9. Ma GW, Griffith TG. Percutaneous repair of acute closed ruptured Achilles tendon: a new technique. Clin Orthop Relat Res 1977;(128):247–55.
10. Fortis AP, Dimas A, Lamprakis AA. Repair of Achilles tendon rupture under endoscopic control. Arthroscopy 2008;24:683–8.
11. Hsu AR, Jones CP, Cohen BE, et al. Clinical outcomes and complications of percutaneous Achilles repair system versus open technique for acute Achilles tendon ruptures. Foot Ankle Int 2015;36:1279–86.
12. Calder JD, Saxby TS. Independent evaluation of a recently described Achilles tendon repair technique. Foot Ankle Int 2006;27:93–6.
13. Maffulli N. Rupture of the Achilles tendon. J Bone Joint Surg Am 1999;81:1019–36.
14. Halasi T, Tallay A, Berkes I. Percutaneous Achilles tendon repair with and without endoscopic control. Knee Surg Sports Traumatol Arthrosc 2003;11:409–14.
15. Turgut A, Gunal I, Maralcan G, et al. Endoscopy, assisted percutaneous repair of the Achilles tendon ruptures: a cadaveric and clinical study. Knee Surg Sports Traumatol Arthrosc 2002;10:130–3.
16. Tang KL, Thermann H, Dai G, et al. Arthroscopically assisted percutaneous repair of fresh closed Achilles tendon rupture by Kessler's suture. Am J Sports Med 2007;35:589–96.
17. Doral MN, Bozkurt M, Turhan E, et al. Percutaneous suturing of the ruptured Achilles tendon with endoscopic control. Arch Orthop Trauma Surg 2009;129:1093–101.
18. Chiu CH, Yeh WL, Tsai MC, et al. Endoscopy-assisted percutaneous repair of acute Achilles tendon tears. Foot Ankle Int 2013;34:1168–76.
19. Huri G, Bicer OS, Ozgozen L, et al. A novel repair method for the treatment of acute Achilles tendon rupture with minimally invasive approach using button implant: a biomechanical study. Foot Ankle Surg 2013;19:261–6.
20. Barske HL, DiGiovanni BF, Douglass M, et al. Current concepts review: isolated gastrocnemius contracture and gastrocnemius recession. Foot Ankle Int 2012;33:915–21.
21. Jastifer JR, Marston J. Gastrocnemius contracture in patients with and without foot pathology. Foot Ankle Int 2016;37:1165–70.
22. Tashjian RZ, Appel AJ, Banerjee R, et al. Endoscopic gastrocnemius recession: evaluation in a cadaver model. Foot Ankle Int 2003;24:607–13.
23. Lui TH. Endoscopic gastrocnemius intramuscular aponeurotic recession. Arthrosc Tech 2015;4:e615–8.
24. Pinney SJ, Sangeorzan BJ, Hansen ST Jr. Surgical anatomy of the gastrocnemius recession (Strayer procedure). Foot Ankle Int 2004;25:247–50.
25. Angthong C, Kanitnate S. Dual-portal endoscopic gastrocnemius recession for the treatment of severe posttraumatic equinus deformity: a case series and a review of technical modifications. J Nippon Med Sch 2012;79:198–203.
26. Trevino S, Gibbs M, Panchbhavi V. Evaluation of results of endoscopic gastrocnemius recession. Foot Ankle Int 2005;26:359–64.

27. Yeap EJ, Shamsul SA, Chong KW, et al. Simple two-portal technique for endoscopic gastrocnemius recession: clinical tip. Foot Ankle Int 2011;32:830–3.
28. Saxena A, Widtfeldt A. Endoscopic gastrocnemius recession: preliminary report on 18 cases. J Foot Ankle Surg 2004;43:302–6.
29. DiDomenico LA, Adams HB, Garchar D. Endoscopic gastrocnemius recession for the treatment of gastrocnemius equinus. J Am Podiatr Med Assoc 2005;95: 410–3.
30. Saxena A, Gollwitzer H, Widtfeldt A, et al. Endoscopic gastrocnemius recession as therapy for gastrocnemius equinus. Z Orthop Unfall 2007;145:499–504 [in German].
31. Grady JF, Kelly C. Endoscopic gastrocnemius recession for treating equinus in pediatric patients. Clin Orthop Relat Res 2010;468:1033–8.
32. Schroeder SM. Uniportal endoscopic gastrocnemius recession for treatment of gastrocnemius equinus with a dedicated EGR system with retractable blade. J Foot Ankle Surg 2012;51:714–9.
33. Phisitkul P, Rungprai C, Femino JE, et al. Endoscopic gastrocnemius recession for the treatment of isolated gastrocnemius contracture: a prospective study on 320 consecutive patients. Foot Ankle Int 2014;35:747–56.
34. Thevendran G, Howe LB, Kaliyaperumal K, et al. Endoscopic gastrocnemius recession procedure using a single portal technique: a prospective study of fifty four consecutive patients. Int Orthop 2015;39:1099–107.
35. Roukis TS, Schweinberger MH. Complications associated with uni-portal endoscopic gastrocnemius recession in a diabetic patient population: an observational case series. J Foot Ankle Surg 2010;49:68–70.
36. Paavola M, Kannus P, Paakkala T, et al. Long-term prognosis of patients with Achilles tendinopathy. An observational 8-year follow-up study. Am J Sports Med 2000;28:634–42.
37. Maffulli N, Binfield PM, Moore D, et al. Surgical decompression of chronic central core lesions of the Achilles tendon. Am J Sports Med 1999;27:747–52.
38. Maquirriain J. Endoscopic release of Achilles peritenon. Arthroscopy 1998;14: 182–5.
39. Thermann H, Benetos IS, Panelli C, et al. Endoscopic treatment of chronic mid-portion Achilles tendinopathy: novel technique with short-term results. Knee Surg Sports Traumatol Arthrosc 2009;17:1264–9.
40. Maquirriain J, Ayerza M, Costa-Paz M, et al. Endoscopic surgery in chronic Achilles tendinopathies: a preliminary report. Arthroscopy 2002;18:298–303.
41. Morag G, Maman E, Arbel R. Endoscopic treatment of hindfoot pathology. Arthroscopy 2003;19:E13.
42. Vega J, Cabestany JM, Golano P, et al. Endoscopic treatment for chronic Achilles tendinopathy. Foot Ankle Surg 2008;14:204–10.
43. Lui TH. Treatment of chronic noninsertional Achilles tendinopathy with endoscopic Achilles tendon debridement and flexor hallucis longus transfer. Foot Ankle Spec 2012;5:195–200.
44. Pearce CJ, Carmichael J, Calder JD. Achilles tendinoscopy and plantaris tendon release and division in the treatment of non-insertional Achilles tendinopathy. Foot Ankle Surg 2012;18:124–7.
45. Maquirriain J. Surgical treatment of chronic Achilles tendinopathy: long-term results of the endoscopic technique. J Foot Ankle Surg 2013;52:451–5.
46. Sammarco GJ, Taylor AL. Operative management of Haglund's deformity in the nonathlete: a retrospective study. Foot Ankle Int 1998;19:724–9.

47. van Dijk CN, van Dyk GE, Scholten PE, et al. Endoscopic calcaneoplasty. Am J Sports Med 2001;29:185–9.
48. Jerosch J, Nasef NM. Endoscopic calcaneoplasty–rationale, surgical technique, and early results: a preliminary report. Knee Surg Sports Traumatol Arthrosc 2003;11:190–5.
49. Leitze Z, Sella EJ, Aversa JM. Endoscopic decompression of the retrocalcaneal space. J Bone Joint Surg Am 2003;85-A:1488–96.
50. Jerosch J, Schunck J, Sokkar SH. Endoscopic calcaneoplasty (ECP) as a surgical treatment of Haglund's syndrome. Knee Surg Sports Traumatol Arthrosc 2007; 15:927–34.
51. Ortmann FW, McBryde AM. Endoscopic bony and soft-tissue decompression of the retrocalcaneal space for the treatment of Haglund deformity and retrocalcaneal bursitis. Foot Ankle Int 2007;28:149–53.
52. Jerosch J, Sokkar S, Ducker M, et al. Endoscopic calcaneoplasty (ECP) in Haglund's syndrome. Indication, surgical technique, surgical findings and results. Z Orthop Unfall 2012;150:250–6 [in German].
53. Kondreddi V, Gopal RK, Yalamanchili RK. Outcome of endoscopic decompression of retrocalcaneal bursitis. Indian J Orthop 2012;46:659–63.
54. Wu Z, Hua Y, Li Y, et al. Endoscopic treatment of Haglund's syndrome with a three portal technique. Int Orthop 2012;36:1623–7.
55. Kaynak G, Ogut T, Yontar NS, et al. Endoscopic calcaneoplasty: 5-year results. Acta Orthop Traumatol Turc 2013;47:261–5.
56. Wong J, Barrass V, Maffulli N. Quantitative review of operative and nonoperative management of Achilles tendon ruptures. Am J Sports Med 2002;30:565–75.
57. Gossage W, Kohls-Gatzoulis J, Solan M. Endoscopic assisted repair of chronic Achilles tendon rupture with flexor hallucis longus augmentation. Foot Ankle Int 2010;31:343–7.
58. Lui TH, Chan WC, Maffulli N. Endoscopic flexor hallucis longus tendon transfer for chronic Achilles tendon rupture. Sports Med Arthrosc 2016;24:38–41.
59. Gedam PN, Rushnaiwala FM. Endoscopy-assisted Achilles tendon reconstruction with a central turndown flap and semitendinosus augmentation. Foot Ankle Int 2016;37:1333–42.
60. Piontek T, Bakowski P, Ciemniewska-Gorzela K, et al. Minimally invasive, endoscopic Achilles tendon reconstruction using semitendinosus and gracilis tendons with Endobutton stabilization. BMC Musculoskelet Disord 2016;17:247.

What Do You Do With The Achilles if You Have No Fancy Toys?

Rajiv Shah, MS[a,b,c,d,e,f,]*, Sampat Dumbre Patil, DNB (Orth)[c,g]

KEYWORDS

- Achilles tendon • Flexor hallucis longus • Semitendinosus tendon • Bony anchorage
- Chronic Achilles rupture

KEY POINTS

- Surgical management of Achilles disorders warrants thorough excision of the degenerated tendon and removal of all impinging bone. Resulting defects can be bridged by various methods like tendon mobilization, V-Y advancement, central turn-down, or tendon transfer.
- Although the flexor hallucis longus is the most commonly used tendon for transfer, large defects in cases of chronic Achilles ruptures may be bridged by use of a distant donor tendon, such as the semitendinosus tendon.
- Bony anchorage of a lengthened or transferred tendon into the calcaneus can be done either with suture anchors or with interference screws.
- In developing countries, such costly implants may not always be available or affordable. This necessitates the adoption of innovative ways to anchor tendons into calcaneus.

INTRODUCTION

The surgical management of insertional and noninsertional Achilles disorders are comprised of 2 key steps. Step 1 is the thorough excision of all necrotic and degenerated tendon and removal of all impinging bony prominences.[1,2] This may result in a tendon defect, which is bridged with various procedures depending upon the size of the defect.[1–3] Defects up to 2 cm can easily be bridged by Achilles tendon mobilization and by pulling the tendon down with the help of traction sutures placed

The authors have nothing to disclose.
a Global Foot and Ankle Council; b Asia-Pacific Foot and Ankle Council; c Indian Foot and Ankle Society; d Sunshine Global Hospitals, Vadodara, Gujarat, India; e Sunshine Global Hospitals, Bharuch, Gujarat, India; f Sunshine Global Hospitals, Surat, Gujarat, India; g Director, Department of Orthopedics, Noble Hospital, Magarpatta, Hadapsar, Pune 411013, Maharashtra, India
* Corresponding author. Department of Orthopaedics, Sunshine Global Hospital, Near Shreyas School, Manjalpur, Vadodara 3900011, India.
E-mail address: rajivortho@gmail.com

Foot Ankle Clin N Am 22 (2017) 801–818
http://dx.doi.org/10.1016/j.fcl.2017.07.008
foot.theclinics.com

in the tendon end (picture 5). Defects up to 2 to 5 cm can be bridged by a V-Y advancement or a central turn down procedure. Defects beyond 5 cm require a tendon transfer, which can be local or distant. The flexor hallucis longus tendon is the most commonly used local tendon transfer. Autogenous semitendinosus is also used as a distant transfer for large defects when allografts are not available.[4]

Step 2 is the bony anchorage of a lengthened/augmented original or transferred tendon to calcaneus. Traditionally this is done either with the use of suture anchors or an interference screw.[5,6] These implants may not be available in developing countries. If available, they may not always be affordable to most of the patients.[7] This requires the use of innovative ways to carry out bony anchorage of tendon.[7] The authors describe their innovative techniques to deal with bony anchorage of tendons without the use of expensive implants.

INDICATIONS

All surgically managed noninsertional and insertional Achilles disorders and chronic Achilles rupture cases (6 weeks after injury) requiring either reattachment of a lengthened Achilles tendon to the calcaneus or requiring attachment of transferred tendons like the flexor hallucis longus (FHL) and semitendinosus to the calcaneus are indications for these procedures. For chronic Achilles ruptures, only patients who complain of significant weakness in daily activities are candidates for surgery. The common feature for all these cases is the lack of availability of expensive implants for bony anchorage of tendon.

CONTRAINDICATIONS

Cases with peripheral vascular disease, peripheral neuropathy, and poor soft tissue envelope are contraindications for these procedures.[2,8] For the chronic Achilles rupture group, patients older than 60 years of age and diabetics are considered as surgical contraindications.[4]

PREOPERATIVE PLANNING

Before surgery, the extent of tendon degeneration is evaluated clinically and radiologically. On radiographs, the presence of an insertional spur and the prominence of a posterosuperior angle of the calcaneus (Haglund deformity) can be diagnosed. Use of ultrasound and MRI also helps in identification of possible extent of tendon degeneration.[1,3,8] A rough estimate is made about the size of tendon defect to remain at the end of tendon debridement and bone removal. A plan is made to bridge the tendon defect and for bony anchorage of the tendon to calcaneus.

SURGICAL PROCEDURE

Surgical procedures will differ depending upon the clinical situations, like treatment of Achilles disorders with reattachment of original or augmented tendon, with local FHL transfer or with distant semitendinosus transfer.

Bone Tunnel-Assisted Bony Anchorage of Achilles Tendon to Calcaneus (for Defects up to 2 or 2–5 cm)

Position
The patient is positioned prone with both the ankles hanging out of operative table. Both of the lower limbs are prepared and draped (**Fig. 1**). This positioning helps in

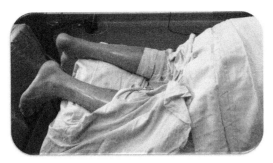

Fig. 1. Prone operative position of patient with preparation of both the lower limbs. Both the ankles are brought out of the table for easy maneuvering of the ankle.

maneuvering of the affected ankle. It also helps in assessment of tendon tension.[1,3] The limb is exsanguinated, and a thigh tourniquet is inflated.

Approach

A straight midline posterior incision extends upwards from Achilles insertion up to 7 cm (**Fig. 2**). The incision may be extended more proximally depending upon the preoperative evaluation of the extent of tendon pathology. Distally, the incision is extended to such a level that complete visualization of tendon insertion and the insertional spur is obtained. The skin and tendon sheath are incised together without creating any plane between them. Distal dissection must be beyond the tendon insertion. The Achilles is vertically split in the midline up to its insertion. The tendon is released both medially and laterally at its insertion to result in a medial and lateral tendon flap.

Bone removal

The insertional bony spur is sharply excised or removed. A self-retaining retractor is placed inside the split tendon, which exposes the retrocalcaneal bursa and the posterosuperior calcaneus prominence (Haglund deformity). The bursa is completely excised. The Haglund deformity is excised with the use of a straight osteotome, taking care to avoid entering a subtalar joint. The clinical picture at this juncture must look without any offending bony projections (**Fig. 3**).At this juncture, image check is done to confirm the adequacy of bone removal (**Fig. 4**).

Tendon excision

The tendon is inspected and palpated for areas of degeneration. Thorough excision of all necrotic tendon and calcifications is carried out until healthy-looking tendon is found. The assessment of the tendon defect is done at this juncture.

Management of defect up to 2 cm

In a case with a defect up to 2 cm, with 2 vertically split tendon flaps, a number 2 Ethibond suture is passed from the distal end of the medial tendon flap. The suture goes upwards in a crisscross manner to suture both medial and lateral tendon flaps together. The suture is then brought down and out to exit from the opposite lateral tendon flap. Standing at the end of the table, an assistant gives continuous tension through the sutures for 5 minutes. This removes all of the slack in the tendon and will close the defect. If required, to gain more length, proximal mobilization

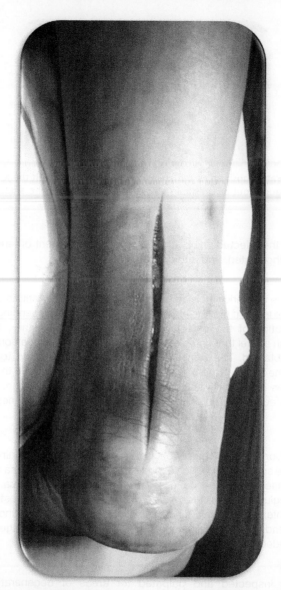

Fig. 2. Posterior vertical midline approach.

of the tendon from its sheath can be done. With the closure of the defect, the 2 tendon flaps with sutures at their ends are ready to be anchored to the bone (**Fig. 5**) The bony anchorage of tendon can be done in different ways, as will be described.

Management of defect up to 2 to 5 cm

V-Y advancement is planned for bridging such a defect. The incision in the skin and tendon sheath needs to be extended upwards up to the musculotendinous junction. The limbs of the V incision in the gastrocnemius fascia are planned and marked as

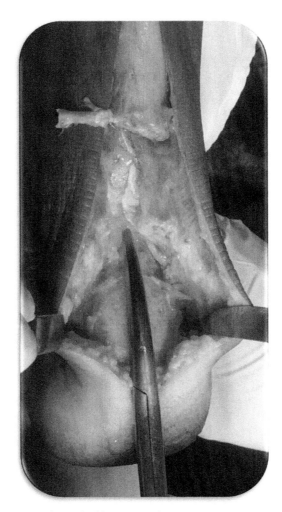

Fig. 3. Clinical picture at the end of bone resection.

double the size of the defect (**Fig. 6**). While carrying out the incision in the gastrocnemius fascia, care is taken to prevent injury to the underlying muscle belly. Tag sutures are passed through the end of the tendon flap. Standing at the end of the table, an assistant gives continuous traction over the tag sutures for 5 minutes. This maneuver gains required length and closes the defect. If required, to gain more length, proximal mobilization of tendon from its sheath can be done. Once the defect is closed, the proximal V incisions in the tendon sheath are closed to make it Y (**Fig. 7**A, B). Tag sutures are replaced with Bunnell sutures with the use of number 2 Ethibond. With sutures out at the distal end of tendon stump, the tendon is ready to be anchored to bone (**Fig. 8**). The bony anchorage of tendon can be done in different ways, as will be described.

Bony anchorage
Bony anchorage of the tendon is done with the formation of 2 parallel bone tunnels in the calcaneus at its original Achilles insertion site. The distance between the 2 bone

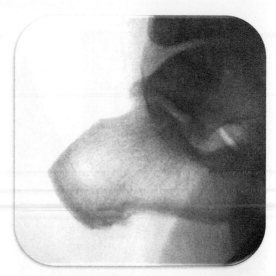

Fig. 4. Intraoperative radiological projection at the end of bone resection.

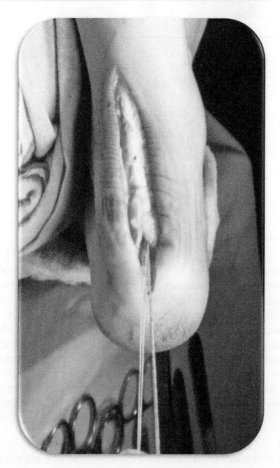

Fig. 5. Sutures brought out from both of the Achilles tendon flaps for bony anchorage.

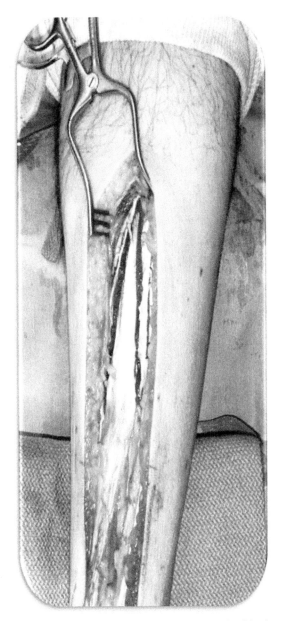

Fig. 6. Limbs of V are marked in gastrocnemius aponeurosis as double the size of the defect to be bridged.

tunnels is at least 2 cm to prevent breakage of intervening bone (**Fig. 9**). The bone tunnels are created with 2 parallel 1.8 mm k-wires. The K-wires are driven in a posterior-to-anterior direction. The K-wires are directed in such a manner that anteriorly they exit through the superior surface of calcaneus (**Fig. 10**). This formulates a strong bone bite between the entry and exit for a strong bony anchorage. K-wires are

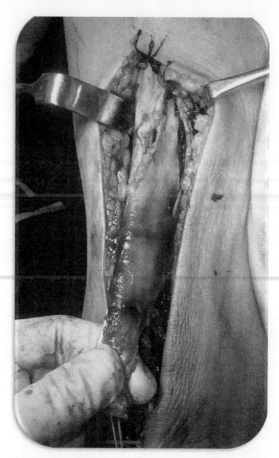

Fig. 7. Sutures brought out from Achilles tendon following V-Y advancement for bony anchorage.

replaced with number 18 hypodermic needles, passed from posterior to anterior in direction. Sutures are threaded out posteriorly through the hypodermic needles. The sutures are pulled tight and are tied with each other over the posterior calcaneus with the ankle in neutral position (**Fig. 11**A, B).

Closure
After lavage, the sheath is closed with absorbable sutures. The skin automatically gets approximated once the sheath is closed and is sutured with nylon. A below-knee plaster slab in a neutral position is given for 4 weeks.

Bone Tunnel Assisted Bony Anchorage of Flexor Hallucis Longus to Calcaneus (for Defect More than 5 cm)

Position
The patient is positioned prone with both of the ankles hanging off of the table for easy maneuvering of the limbs. Both the lower limbs are prepared and draped. A tourniquet is inflated after exsanguination of the limb.

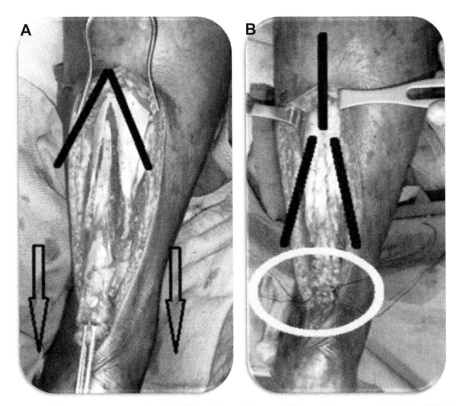

Fig. 8. (*A*) Gastrocnemius fascial V incision being pulled, at closure of defect (*B*) it becomes Y.

Exposure

Exposure is carried out with a straight posterior incision that extends upwards from the Achilles insertion up to 7 cm proximally. The skin and sheath are incised together without creating a plane between the two. The lower extent of the incision and dissection must expose the Achilles insertion and insertional spur fully.

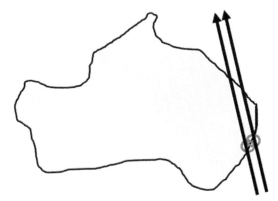

Fig. 9. Diagrammatic representation showing side view of location and direction of vertical bone tunnels in calcaneus.

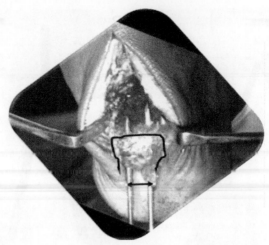

Fig. 10. Intraoperative picture showing direction and spacing of 2 vertical bone tunnels in calcaneus.

Excision of bone and tendon

The procedures are the same as those previously described for insertional and non-insertional Achilles disorders. All degenerated and calcified tendon areas, together with all impinging bone, are thoroughly excised. If the resultant tendon defect is more than 5 cm, a transfer of the flexor hallucis longus is planned. The authors prefer a short harvest of the FHL.

Flexor hallucis longus harvest

The Achilles stump is retracted proximally to expose the fascia of the posterior compartment. The muscle belly of the FHL underlying this fascia is identified. A vertical cut in the fascia is made to expose the FHL muscle belly and is traced distally up to the tendon. The tendon is gently hooked out with mixture forceps (**Fig. 12**).

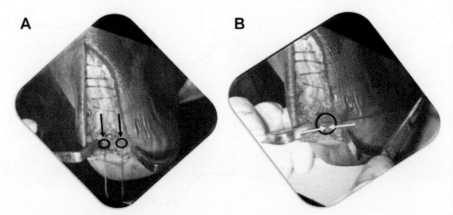

Fig. 11. (*A*) Passage of sutures through the bone tunnels for anchorage of vertically slit Achilles tendon. (*B*) Final bone tunnel anchorage of the Achilles tendon.

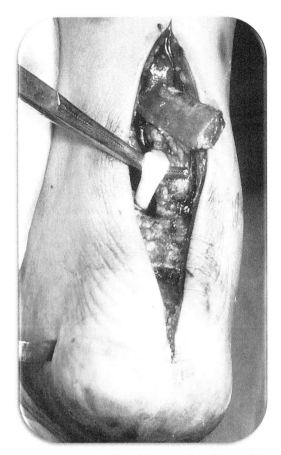

Fig. 12. Posterior fascia is cut, and tendon of flexor hallucis longus is hooked out.

Identification of the tendon is assisted by simultaneous movements of the great toe.[3] The tendon is freed from all the sides starting proximally and going as distally as possible to gain maximum length. With the maximal plantar flexion of the great toe and the ankle, and with maximum pull over the tendon by an assistant, the tendon is released as distally as possible. The knife cut is directed from medial to lateral to prevent injury to surrounding neurovascular structures. Holding sutures through the harvested FHL tendon may be applied for easy maneuverability of the tendon (**Fig. 13**). The tendon is now ready for bony anchorage.

Bony anchorage of flexor hallucis longus tendon

Bony anchorage of the FHL tendon is done with the help of 2 parallel and transverse bone tunnels drilled through the calcaneus. Bone tunnels are created with the help of 2 1.8 mm k-wires that are drilled transversely through the calcaneus starting medially and exiting laterally. The distance between the anterior and posterior bone tunnels is kept at minimum of 2 cm (**Fig. 14**). Bone tunnels are positioned in such a manner that good bone bite is maintained all around the tunnels to prevent bone breakage at suturing (**Fig. 15**). A hypodermic needle number 18 replaces the k-wire in the posterior most tunnel (**Fig. 16**). The suture ends are, turn by

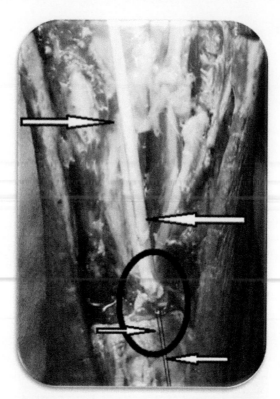

Fig. 13. Holding sutures tied at the end of the tendon of flexor halluces longus to pull the tendon.

turn, threaded with the help of the hypodermic needle to exit medially and laterally. The medial and lateral arm of the sutures are tied with each other in the center with tension. The ankle is in neutral position during tendon tensioning. With the help of the hypodermic needle number 18, a number 2 Ethibond is threaded transversely through the anterior tunnel. Sutures are passed through the tendon and tied to each other in the center. These sutures lie anterior to already anchored tendon. Resultant transfer now has a solid double anchorage with good tendon tension (**Fig. 17**). The proximal Achilles stump is pulled and sutured with the muscle belly of the FHL with 2 absorbable sutures on both sides. This provides strength and additional blood supply to the transfer.[1–3]

Closure
After lavage, the sheath is closed with absorbable sutures. The skin gets approximated once the sheath is closed and sutured with nylon. A below-knee plaster slab in a neutral position is given for 4 weeks.

Bone Tunnel-Assisted Bony Anchorage of Semitendinosus to Calcaneus (for Defects More than 5 cm)

Position
The patient is positioned prone, and both of the lower limbs are prepared and draped.

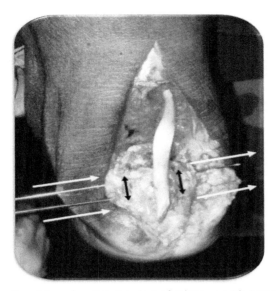

Fig. 14. Intraoperative picture showing top view of calcaneus with 2 transverse bone tunnels with direction and spacing of k-wires.

Incision & preparation

A vertical midline incision centering over the palpable gap is taken and deepened with sharp dissection (**Fig. 18**). Thorough debridement of the tendon ends, and intervening fibrous tissue is done. The gap between the 2 tendon ends is measured in neutral position of ankle. If the defect is more than 5 cm, the semitendinosus tendon is harvested from the same leg and used for reconstruction.

Graft harvest

For harvesting the semitendinosus tendon, the knee is flexed, and a 3 to 4 cm incision medial to the tibial tuberosity is taken (**Fig. 19**A, B). The tendon is prepared using

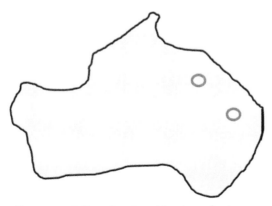

Fig. 15. Diagrammatic representation showing side view of calcaneus with location and spacing of transverse bone tunnels.

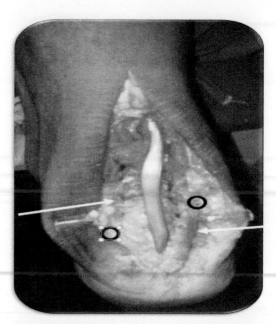

Fig. 16. Intraoperative picture showing short harvest of flexor hallucis longus tendon with 2 hypodermic needles passed through transverse bone tunnels in calcaneus.

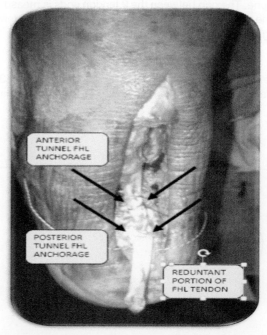

Fig. 17. Flexor hallucis longus transfer fixed with sutures through posterior and anterior transverse bone tunnels in calcaneus.

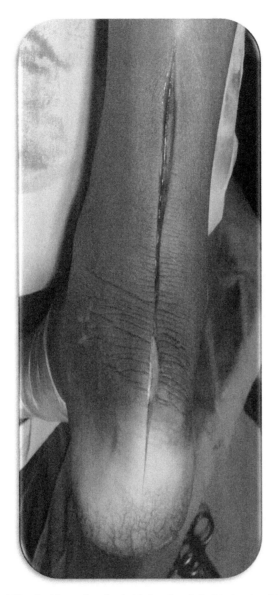

Fig. 18. Vertical midline incision taken for bridging the defect in tendoachilles with semitendinosus tendon.

number 2 Ethibond. Attention is given to prepare the ends of the graft that will facilitate the passage of graft through the tunnel in the calcaneus.

Bony anchorage
A transverse tunnel in the calcaneus is drilled over a guide wire, which is directed from medial to lateral (**Fig. 20**) at about 1.5 cm below the point of insertion of Achilles tendon (**Fig. 21**). A 4.5 mm cannulated drill is used over the guide wire, and then the

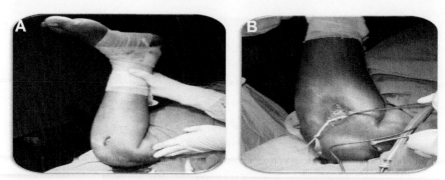

Fig. 19. (*A*) Incision medial to tibial tuberosity for harvest of semitendinosus. (*B*) Semitendinosus graft harvested through with knee in flexion with patient in prone position.

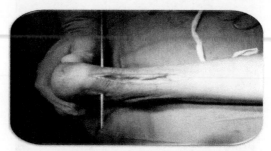

Fig. 20. Transverse tunnel in calcaneum drilled with 4.5 mm cannulated drill over a guide-wire passed from medial to lateral side, 1.5 cm below the attachment of the Achilles tendon.

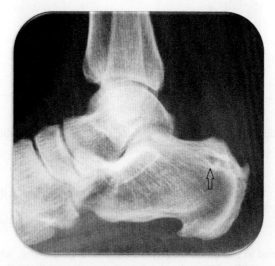

Fig. 21. Lateral radiograph of the ankle joint showing position of the calcaneal tunnel for passage of semitendinosus tendon transfer.

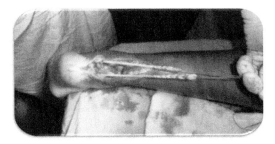

Fig. 22. The semitendinosus graft passed through calcaneus and then taken upward to pass through the proximal end of Achilles.

graft is passed through the tunnel. Proximally, the graft is passed through the debrided tendon end and then sutured to itself (**Fig. 22**). The suturing of graft to itself and Achilles tendon side to side will avoid the sliding of the tendon in the tunnel (**Fig. 23**). This technique has resulted in satisfactory postoperative results (**Fig. 24**).

POSTOPERATIVE CARE

A below-knee plaster slab in a neutral position is given for 4 weeks. Sutures are removed at the end of 10 days. Nonweight-bearing mobilization of ankle is started after removal of the plaster splint. Mobilization and strengthening exercises follow. The patient starts ambulation over a period of the next 2 weeks after gaining adequate strength and range of motion.

COMPLICATIONS AND MANAGEMENT

Specific to the bony anchorage of the tendon, the most common complication is the breakage or fracture of intervening bone or bone tunnel. This is better prevented than managed. Spacing between the 2 tunnels and the location of the tunnels must be so that there is a good intervening and surrounding bone. If the tunnel breaks, the option of creating another tunnel by the side of the same tunnel remains. Failure with transverse tunnel can also be managed with use of additional vertical tunnel and vice versa. A hypersensitivity reaction to Ethibond suture material resulting in a sinus formation is common. It usually settles down once the offending suture is removed under local anesthesia.

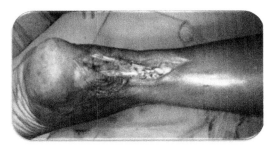

Fig. 23. The graft is sutured to itself and with the Achilles side to side.

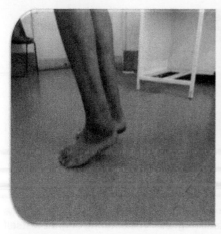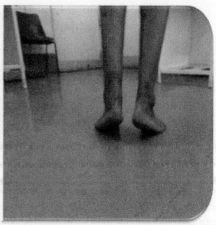

Fig. 24. The postoperative clinical picture showing final result.

SUMMARY

Reattachment of either the original tendon or a transferred tendon does not always necessitate use of fancy implants like interference screws or suture anchors. Given a case where these implants are not available, bony anchorage of tendons can easily be done with the use of bone tunnels. Bone tunnels could be transverse or vertical depending upon the case. Tunnels drilled parallel with adequate surrounding bone would be success denominator. Two tunnels give better anchorage strength. Bone tunnel anchorage of tendon is user-friendly, cost-effective, and safe with reproducible good end results. The technique is a boon for developing countries, where fancy gadgets are either not available or not affordable.

REFERENCES

1. Steven KN, Daniel CF. Tendon transfers in the treatment of Achilles' tendon disorders. Foot Ankle Clin N Am 2014;19:73–98.
2. Vinod KP. Percutaneous techniques for tendon transfers in the foot and ankle. Foot Ankle Clin 2014;19:113–22.
3. Wapner KL, Pavlock GS, Hecht PJ, et al. Repair of chronic Achilles tendon rupture with flexor halluces longus tendon transfer. Foot Ankle 1993;14:443–9.
4. Dumbre Patil SS, Dumbre Patil DP, Basa VR, et al. Semitendinosus tendon autograft for reconstruction of large defects in chronic Achilles tendon ruptures. Foot Ankle Int 2014;35(7):699–705.
5. Maffulli N, Testa V, Capasso G, et al. Calcific insertional Achilles tendinopathy. Replacement with bone anchors. Am J Sports Med 2004;32:174–82.
6. Cottom JM, Hyer CF, Berlet GC, et al. Flexor hallucis tendon transfer with an interference screw for chronic Achilles tendinosis: a report of 62 cases. Foot Ankle Spec 2008;1(5):280–7.
7. Rajiv S. Indian foot and ankle scenario. Foot Ankle Spec 2011;4:390–5.
8. Panchbhavi VK. Chronic Achilles tendon repair with flexor hallucis longus tendon harvested using a minimally invasive technique. Tech Foot Ankle Surg 2007;6(2):123–9.

Treatment of Acute and Chronic Tibialis Anterior Tendon Rupture and Tendinopathy

CrossMark

Elizabeth Harkin, MD*, Michael Pinzur, MD, Adam Schiff, MD

KEYWORDS

- Anterior tibial tendon • Tendon rupture • Repair • Reconstruction

KEY POINTS

- Rupture of the tibialis anterior tendon is a rare injury that has primarily been studied through case reports and low-volume case studies.
- Common mechanisms of injury include direct trauma, closed indirect trauma, an applied dorsiflexion force, and spontaneous rupture.
- The site of spontaneous rupture corresponds with an avascular zone beneath the inferior and superior extensor retinaculum.
- Patients typically present with signs and symptoms including anterior ankle pain, a palpable tendon defect, drop-foot gait, and decreased dorsiflexion strength.
- Further studies are needed to evaluate the comparative efficacy of primary repair, tendon transfer, and autograft and allograft reconstruction.

INTRODUCTION

Although injury to the tibialis anterior (TA) tendon is rare, it is still the third most common tendon rupture of the lower extremity after Achilles and patellar tendon ruptures.[1] These injuries are mainly described in the literature through small case series and individual case reports. Classically there are 2 described mechanisms of injury: (1) spontaneous rupture in an elderly patient following a plantarflexion eversion injury resulting in a drop-foot gait; and (2) open or direct trauma in a young, active patient. Nonoperative and operative treatment options have been described based on patient age and activity level. Surgical treatment options include direct repair, tendon transfer, or free tendon autograft and allograft reconstruction based on injury chronicity and the size of the tendon defect.

Disclosure: Dr A. Schiff is a consultant for Stryker, Sonoma, RTI. Dr M. Pinzur is a consultant for Stryker and Wright Medical (Biomimetics). Dr E. Harkin has an immediate family member that is a paid employee of Globus Medical.

Department of Orthopaedic Surgery and Rehabilitation, Loyola University Medical Center, 2160 South First Avenue, Maguire Suite 1700, Maywood, IL 60153, USA
* Corresponding author.
E-mail address: elizabeth.harkin@lumc.edu

Foot Ankle Clin N Am 22 (2017) 819–831
http://dx.doi.org/10.1016/j.fcl.2017.07.009

ANATOMY

The TA tendon acts primarily to dorsiflex the ankle and invert the foot. It allows controlled plantar flexion via eccentric loading during the heel strike phase of gait and dorsiflexion via concentric loading during the swing phase of gait.[2] The TA muscle belly originates from the proximal half of the anterior tibia, lower lateral tibial condyle, lateral tibia, and interosseous membrane. The muscle transitions at the musculocutaneous junction to become more tendinous, covered by a synovial sheath, before coursing beneath the superior and inferior extensor retinaculum. There are 3 described variations of insertion onto the medial border of the medial cuneiform and base of the first metatarsal: wide slip on the cuneiform and narrow slip on the first metatarsal, 2 slips of equal width, and a wide slip on the first metatarsal and a narrow slip on the medial cuneiform.[1] Proximally the blood supply to the tendon is provided by the anterior tibial artery and distally it is supplied by branches of the medial tarsal artery. Blood vessels penetrate the tendon via viniculae from the peritenon to create anastomoses that travel longitudinally in an intratendinous network. Posteriorly the tendon has a complete vascular network from the musculocutaneous junction to insertion; however, anteriorly there is an avascular zone 4.5 to 6.7 cm in length that correlates with the most common sites of spontaneous rupture.[3] Innervation to the muscle and tendon is supplied by the deep peroneal nerve.

TENDINOSIS

Tendinosis of the TA tendon is typically seen in overweight women with medial foot pain that is worse at night or as an overuse injury in athletes presenting with anterior ankle pain following an increase in activity.[4,5] On examination, patients have swelling and discrete tenderness at the insertion of the TA tendon. Patients describe pain with resisted dorsiflexion. Tendinosis can be differentiated from a tendon rupture by the preservation of dorsiflexion strength and the absence of a drop-foot gait pattern, as well as the absence of a palpable tendon defect. The TA passive stretch test is a provocative maneuver for TA tendinosis that results in reproduction of pain with ankle plantarflexion, hindfoot eversion, midfoot abduction, and an applied pronation force with sensitivity of 90% and specificity of 95%.[4] Classic MRI findings include a thickened TA tendon with possible longitudinal tears, peritendon edema, and synovitis **(Fig. 1)**.

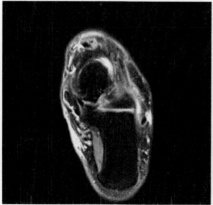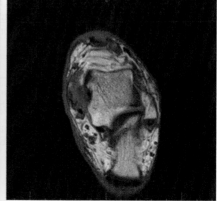

Fig. 1. MRI showing tendinosis of the anterior tibial tendon.

Repetitive trauma and chronic inflammation result in increased tendon vascularity and myxoid degeneration of the tendon interstitium. Standard treatment is nonoperative symptomatic management via immobilization with an ankle-foot orthosis (AFO) to hold the ankle in a plantigrade position. For the few cases that fail nonoperative management, longitudinal tears and loss of fibrillary structure may contribute to the lack of response to conservative treatment. In resistant cases, surgical management may be considered. Grundy and colleagues[6] reported good outcomes with debridement, repair with suture anchor fixation, and augmentation with adjacent tendon transfer in cases with greater than 50% tendon involvement.

CLINICAL PRESENTATION FOR ACUTE AND CHRONIC TENDON RUPTURE

Most patients report an insidious onset. Less commonly, patients report an acute episode or some form of indirect trauma. Case reports have described an association between spontaneous rupture and underlying degenerative processes such as inflammatory arthritis, psoriasis, systemic lupus erythematosus, hyperparathyroidism, rheumatoid arthritis, gout, impingement from exostosis, local steroid injection, diabetes, poliomyelitis, and other spinal cord injuries.[1,7–9] In cases of direct trauma, the tendon is at risk because it lies over the distal surface of the tibia and is therefore exposed in the setting of fractures or anterior lacerations. The classic mechanism of acute rupture occurs with supination of the ankle joint and an applied abrupt plantar flexion force against resistance.[10] Several studies have shown that the location of the most frequent site of spontaneous rupture is within 5 and 30 mm from the tendon insertion, which correlates with an avascular zone in which the tendon courses beneath the superior and inferior extensor retinaculum.[4,8] Acute tendon rupture commonly occurs in young patients following trauma or high-functional-level activity. Patients present with acute onset of severe pain and swelling to the dorsum of the foot and ankle after a specific moment of rupture. Chronic tendon ruptures more commonly occur in elderly patients and diabetics with a history of gait problems, lack of coordination, catching of the foot on irregular or uneven ground, and painless drop foot with little or no antecedent trauma. A delay in presentation or diagnosis of chronic tendon ruptures can occur as the extensor hallucis longus (EHL) and extensor digitorum longus (EDL) can compensate as weak dorsiflexors. Markarian and colleagues[11] found that, on average, presentation after chronic tendon ruptures is delayed 10 weeks. In cases of chronic tendon rupture, patients may go on to develop a mild progressive flatfoot deformity, Achilles contracture, or clawing of the toes as the EHL and EDL attempt to compensate for loss of function.[12]

PHYSICAL EXAMINATION

On physical examination, it is important to analyze the patient's gait for slapping of the foot caused by insufficient dorsiflexion and supination resulting in an inability to clear the floor during swing phase. Significant to minimal foot drop may also be present secondary to uncontrolled plantarflexion. Inspection for anterior ankle swelling and palpation of the tendon along its distribution are needed, noting any tenderness, defect, or fixed mass that may indicate a ruptured and retracted tendon (**Fig. 2**).

Provocative testing shows decreased range of motion and dorsiflexion strength of the foot and first ray compared with the contralateral side. According to Otte and colleagues,[10] 80% of dorsiflexion force across the ankle is produced by the TA and the remaining weak dorsiflexion force is preserved by the pull of the EHL and EDL. Secondarily this may result in increased eversion during dorsiflexion secondary to the unopposed pull of the peroneals. With consideration for the patient's baseline

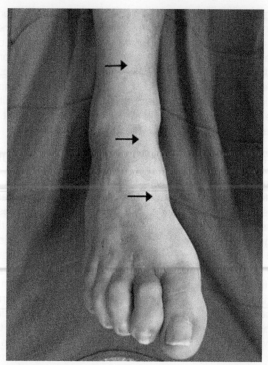

Fig. 2. The course of the anterior tibial tendon. *Arrows* outlining the anatomic course of the anterior tibial tendon.

functional status, more dynamic maneuvers, including the inability to walk on the heels, also indicate weakness.

IMAGING STUDIES

As with any injury to the foot and ankle, weight-bearing radiographs are necessary to rule out any other disorder; however, the diagnosis is primarily based on clinical examination. Ultrasonography is a useful tool to evaluate the dynamic function of any tendon within its sheath. An MRI scan can be obtained to identify a tendon rupture or incomplete tear, particularly in patients without any antecedent trauma. On MRI, disorder and tendon rupture is indicated by gapping and focal high signal intensity compared with surrounding tissues (**Fig. 3**). This finding should be differentiated from tendinosis, in which a thickened tendon with surrounding synovitis is observed.

TREATMENT

There is no general consensus for operative versus nonoperative treatment of anterior tibial tendon ruptures. Prospective outcome measurements are limited by the number of case reports and case series cited in the literature. Treatment goals are to relieve pain and improve function with consideration of age, chronicity of the injury, baseline functional capacity, and medical comorbidities. In general, young, active, healthy, and high-functioning patients benefit from operative management. In addition, those who have failed an AFO or have developed an Achilles contracture could benefit from surgical intervention. However, elderly, ill, or low-demand patients can be managed

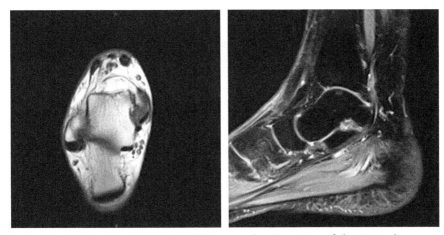

Fig. 3. Axial (*left*) and sagittal (*right*) MRI images showing a tear of the TA tendon.

appropriately with immobilization in an AFO. The chronicity of the injury is also an important factor because ruptures more than 4 weeks old may result in greater tendon retraction, limiting the ability for a direct repair.[2]

NONOPERATIVE TREATMENT

Conservative treatment with an AFO (**Fig. 4**), physical therapy, and activity modification is most appropriate in older, low-demand, sedentary patients. The purpose of the AFO is to prevent the peroneals from pronating the foot and to reduce the weak dorsiflexion force exerted by the EHL and EDL.[13] However, several studies have found that compliance with AFO treatment can be difficult. Ouzounian and Anderson[14] found that 60% of patients treated conservatively refused bracing or found it too restrictive. Patients can anticipate a loss of dorsiflexion strength and motion as the proximal tendon retracts under the extensor retinaculum and becomes adherent to adjacent

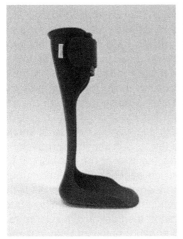
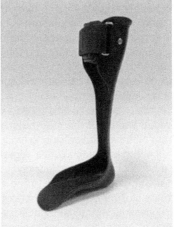

Fig. 4. AFOs used in the nonoperative treatment of anterior tibial tendon injuries.

structures.[11,15] Patients may also experience persistent anterior ankle pain as the EHL and EDL compensate for decreased dorsiflexion strength. Some cases series have also noted a mild progressive pes planus deformity as the peroneals act without opposition to evert and plantarflex the foot causing medial column pronation and midfoot collapse.[13] Patients show an inability to stand on uneven surfaces, slapping gait, increased medial forefoot plantar pressure, frequent ankle sprains, and attenuation of the posterior tibial tendon.[16] Because the Achilles can pull unopposed, equinus contractures can develop. In the author's opinion, bracing, including nocturnal bracing, can help decrease the risk of this equinus. Although these patients may not achieve full functional or gait recovery, these differences do not produce significant limitations in low-demand patients.[11]

SURGICAL MANAGEMENT

For patients who have failed nonoperative management or young, high-demand patients, surgical management is indicated. The chronicity of the injury should also be considered because it affects the degree of retraction and presence of secondary concomitant deformity. In cases of acute laceration or rupture, the tendon can retract beneath the extensor retinaculum and become adherent to nearby structures. Urgent surgical treatment of acute injuries reduces the likelihood of retraction and contracture that might hinder the ability to perform a primary repair. The approach to surgical management in cases of chronic rupture may require bridging of a defect with an adjacent tendon transfer or free graft. In patients with chronic injuries it is important to recognize secondary deformities such as Achilles tendon contractures that would prevent maximum dorsiflexion during repair or reconstruction. Surgical management options for anterior tibial tendon ruptures include primary repair, nonanatomic repair, reconstruction with adjacent tendon transfer, free autograft reconstruction, and allograft reconstruction.

SURGICAL TECHNIQUE FOR PRIMARY REPAIR

In order to perform a primary repair for a ruptured anterior tibial tendon there must be adequate tendon length, mobility, and structure. Primary repair is performed with the patient positioned supine with an anterior curvilinear incision from the first cuneiform to the superior extensor retinaculum. The superficial dissection is directed medial to the EHL and the ends of the tendon are appropriately debrided (**Fig. 5**).

Options for repair include a z-lengthening with side-to-side anastomosis or a direct end-to-end repair using a Bunnell, Krackow, or modified Kessler suture technique.[1] Depending on the level of rupture, a nonanatomic repair may be performed to reconstruct the anterior tibial tendon. In cases of distal rupture or avulsion fracture, the tendon can be reconstructed with a suture anchor in the navicular, first cuneiform, or a horizontal drill hole through which the tendon is passed and then sutured onto itself.[14] In contrast, Sammarco and colleagues[5] described fixation into the medial cuneiform or medial aspect of the first metatarsal base with an additional anchor in the dorsal aspect of the navicular. During closure the tendon sheath is repaired; however, there are differences in techniques regarding the role of the extensor retinaculum following repair. For example, Neumayer and colleagues[17] described supplemental tenodesis of the repaired tendon to the extensor retinaculum to protect the repair and/or primary closure of the extensor retinaculum to restore its pulley effect. However, other investigators advise against repairing the inferior retinaculum to prevent the formation of adhesions while leaving the superior extensor retinaculum intact to prevent bowstringing of the repaired tendon.[2] Postoperatively the repair is protected

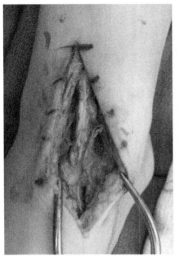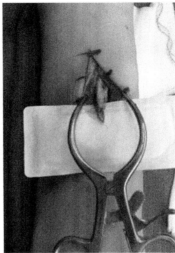

Fig. 5. Superficial dissection exposing an acute anterior tibial tendon tear.

by below-the-knee casting in a neutral position. Several studies have reported decreased plantarflexion strength following primary repair; however, these deficits did not lead to any patient-reported functional deficits.[1,18] A modification to primary repair using an anterior tibial tendon sliding graft can be performed in cases in which tendon retraction has resulted in a 2-cm to 4-cm defect. This technique requires sufficient healthy tendon following debridement of both proximal and distal tendon segments. The proximal tendon is split up to the level of the musculotendinous junction, at which point half the width of the proximal tendon is harvested and transferred distally where it is anastomosed to the proximal and distal tendon segments in an end-to-end repair (**Fig. 6**).[19–21]

SURGICAL TECHNIQUE FOR TENDON TRANSFER RECONSTRUCTION

In cases of tendon defects larger than 4 cm and therefore an inability to perform a primary repair or anterior tibial tendon sliding graft, reconstruction can be performed with an adjacent tendon transfer. Many techniques have been described, including reconstruction with the EHL, EDL, peroneus brevis tendon, and posterior tibial tendon transfer. Perhaps the most commonly described technique is an EHL tendon transfer.[2,22] The EHL tendon is detached from its insertion point on the first metatarsophalangeal joint and is tenodesed to the proximal stump of the TA tendon in a parallel orientation. A variety of techniques have been described for fixation following tenodesis; a bony tunnel can be created for passage of the reconstructed anterior tibial tendon to the navicular, to the first metatarsal base, horizontally or vertically through the medial cuneiform,[3] or the horizontal bony tunnel can be extended from the medial cuneiform through the middle cuneiform and exiting the lateral cuneiform, depending on the length of the EHL graft.[2] The graft is then tensioned with the ankle held in maximal dorsiflexion. Fixation is achieved by either suturing the end of the reconstructed tendon back onto itself or attaching it to the distal stump of the TA tendon,[11] or by using a pull-out wire, bony anchor, or interference screw. In addition, the distal stump of the EHL tendon is tenodesed to the extensor hallucis brevis (EHB) or the EHB is cut and sutured to the distal stump of the EHL. Alternatively, the EDL can also be used

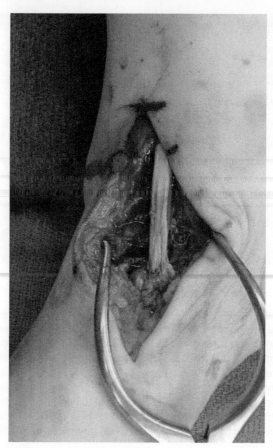

Fig. 6. Primary repair of an acute ATT tear.

to reconstruct a large defect in the anterior tibial tendon using the Kelikian procedure.[23] With this technique, the EDL of the second and third toes is woven through the debrided proximal stump of the anterior tibial tendon at 2 separate points, then it is tenodesed to the EDB.[11] For larger defects, other reconstruction options include peroneus brevis tendon transfer, free tendon autograft, or allograft. In a case report, Forst and colleagues[7] used the peroneus brevis tendon to graft a 9-cm defect in a delayed reconstruction. Subsequently the proximal peroneus brevis stump was anastomosed to the peroneus longus in a side-to-side fashion and the patient did not have a significant pronation deficit. Another option, shown by Pinzur and colleagues,[24] used a combined anterior and posterior tibial tendon reconstruction through the interosseous membrane in the setting of posttraumatic peroneal nerve palsy.

OPTIONS FOR FREE TENDON AUTOGRAFT

In patients in whom adjacent tendon transfer is not available or is insufficient to reconstruct the defect in the debrided TA tendon, a free tendon autograft harvest and reconstruction can be performed. Surgical techniques, including harvesting the peroneus tertius, gracilis, plantaris, Achilles tendon, or semitendinosus, have been described. Similar to reconstruction with tendon transfer, the graft must be tensioned in dorsiflexion and requires fixation with either an interference screw, staple, endobutton, Ethibond, or FiberWire.

In one of the largest case studies of surgical treatment of TA tendon rupture, Sammarco and colleagues[5] used several different repair and reconstruction techniques, including using free tendon autograft harvested from the peroneus tertius tendon, EDL, gracilis, and Achilles tendon. When harvesting the peroneus tertius or EDL, Sammarco and colleagues[5] resected 8 to 10 cm of the tendon and folded the tendon 2 to 3 times to maximize the smaller tendon diameter to bridge defects of less than 3 cm. The remaining free segment of the peroneus tertius or EDL tendon was sutured to the intact extensor digitorum communis (EDC) tendons. Free tendon autograft harvested from the posterior compartment is another viable reconstructive option, although it requires a separate incision and dissection plane. The plantaris tendon can be identified preoperatively on MRI and harvested for reconstruction. If on intraoperative evaluation the plantaris is insufficient, a 4-cm Achilles tendon graft can be harvested through the same incision.[5]

Alternatively, a free gracilis autograft can be harvested from the ipsilateral pes anserinus. Stravrou and colleagues[25] passed the harvested gracilis graft through a bony tunnel created in the medial cuneiform to create a double-stranded graft that was used for an end-to-end reconstruction to the proximal anterior tibial tendon stump. In comparison, Yamazaki and colleagues[26] created a soft tissue tunnel by making a small slit through each of the anterior tibial tendon stumps then folding the graft until it was quadrupled and the ends were bound in a side-to-side fashion. In addition, the reconstruction was reinforced at the entry and exit points of the soft tissue tunnel with multiple sutures between the graft and each anterior tibial tendon stump.

Instead of harvesting the gracilis from the pes anserinus, reconstruction with a semitendinosus autograft is another viable option.[27] Michels and colleagues[28] used semitendinosus autografts in a 12-patient case series with a minimally invasive approach, doubled graft, and biotenodesis screw fixation. In their series, patients tolerated the loss of the semitendinosus tendon without complication and also showed a significant improvement in American Orthopaedic Foot & Ankle Society (AOFAS) scores.

ALLOGRAFT RECONSTRUCTION

Indications for allograft reconstruction for anterior tibial tendon rupture include chronic rupture with retraction, a defect greater than 4 cm, or to prevent the morbidity associated with tendon transfer or autograft reconstruction. Investigators have described several techniques for allograft reconstruction using semitendinosus,[1] gracilis, peroneus longus, anterior tibial tendon,[29] and Achilles tendon allografts.[30] Allografts are available with bone block attachment or free tendon ends, which can be anchored with drill holes or primary suture repair in addition to the hardware options used in autograft fixation. For example, Huh and colleagues[29] performed chronic anterior tibial tendon reconstructions using predominantly anterior tibial tendon allografts for large segmental defects in 11 patients. Patients experienced improved dorsiflexion strength, pain scores, and functional outcomes measured by the Short Form-12 and AOFAS scores.[29] In a case report by Anagnostokos and colleagues,[1] reconstruction of a chronic TA tendon rupture with a large defect was performed using a semitendinosus allograft with only a mild decrease in strength in dorsal extension and plantarflexion strength at 30° 1 year postoperatively compared with the contralateral side. In addition, a case report by Aderinto and Gross[30] used an Achilles tendon allograft for a chronic anterior tibial tendon rupture with a 4-cm defect caused by retraction. At the 8-year follow-up, the patient continued to ambulate independently without pain or deformity. These results show that allograft reconstruction is a safe, reliable option for patients with large defects and that it also avoids any donor site morbidity of tendon transfer and autograft harvest.

AUGMENTATION

It may be necessary to simultaneously address concomitant deformities while performing TA tendon repair or reconstruction. Percutaneous tendoachilles lengthening or gastrocnemius recession can be performed at the time of repair in order to achieve maximal dorsiflexion during graft tensioning, to achieve balance between the flexor and extensor compartments,[12] and to prevent the antagonistic effect of the gastrocnemius during the recovery period in order to protect the repair or reconstruction.[15] According to Sammarco and colleagues,[5] the generally accepted practice is to perform a percutaneous release if 5° of dorsiflexion cannot be achieved with the knee in full extension.[5] Other investigators argue that tendoachilles lengthening or gastrocnemius recession is indicated if there is a 10° to 15° difference compared with contralateral side.[2] In addition, if the presence of an Achilles contracture is noted preoperatively, particularly in the case of chronic tendon rupture, it can be addressed with a preoperative and postoperative stretching program. Eckel and Nunley[31] proposed an alternative method of adjuvant gastrocnemius Botox injection to prevent its antagonistic effect during the recovery period.

POSTOPERATIVE MANAGEMENT

Following repair or reconstruction, the operative limb is traditionally immobilized in a below-the-knee cast in maximal dorsiflexion. The decision of when to allow the patient to begin active range of motion and weight bearing depends on surgeon preference, surgical technique, and baseline patient mobility. Patients are typically progressed to full weight bearing between 3 and 6 weeks postoperatively; however, they remain immobilized in either a walking boot or AFO for up to 12 weeks. Active range of motion is initiated between 6 and 12 weeks postoperatively depending on whether a repair, transfer, or reconstruction was performed. After immobilization, patients can progress from walking to jogging with slow progression into dynamic athletic activities such as jumping, running, and sport-specific movements.

COMPLICATIONS

Similar to nonoperative treatment, possible complications of surgical treatment include decreased dorsiflexion strength, rerupture, and the formation of adhesions between the tendon and extensor retinaculum. However, there are complications inherent in and unique to operative management, such as failure of the repair or reconstruction, wound infection, neuroma formation, entrapment of the intermediate branch of the superficial peroneal nerve, loss of fixation, and/or decreased function at the rupture site and donor site. Because of the low number of reported cases, the incidence of surgical complications cannot be measured but should be part of the discussion with patients considering surgical intervention.

SURGICAL OUTCOMES

Several studies have evaluated the efficacy of operative versus nonoperative treatment of TA tendon ruptures. A classic article by Dooley and colleagues[8] reviewed all reported cases and found that nonoperative patients developed a mild to moderate flatfoot deformity with persistent aching about the ankle, whereas patients who underwent operative management had improved functional outcomes but did not necessarily return to full activity. In a small case series of acute anterior tibial tendon ruptures by Gwynne-Jones and colleagues,[32] 5 patients were treated operatively with either anatomic or nonanatomic repair compared with 2 patients treated nonoperatively. Four of the 5 operative patients returned to activity with no functional limitations, and the mean Foot and Ankle Outcome Score was 85 compared with 52 in the nonoperative group.[32] In one of the largest case studies to date, Ouzounian and Anderson[14] treated 5 patients nonoperatively with an AFO when tolerated and 7 patients with surgical repair or reconstruction. Ten of the 12 patients were allowed to elect to have operative versus nonoperative treatment and, of those who chose operative management, the patients were more physically active, presented earlier following a traumatic event, and were on average 20 years younger.[14] Although no direct comparisons were made, patients treated nonoperatively generally had walking limitations and a drop-foot gait, and patients treated with repair or reconstruction had improved functional ability, increased dorsiflexion strength, nonlimiting loss of ankle motion, and no residual foot drop or pain. From this, the investigators concluded that there are 2 distinctly different clinical presentations of anterior tibialis tendon ruptures and they should be treated accordingly. In contrast, a retrospective study by Markarian and colleagues[11] reviewed the treatment of 8 nonoperative and 8 operative cases treated by anatomic repair, nonanatomic repair, EHL transfer, or EDC transfer. Average follow-up of 3.86 and 6.68 years respectively showed no statistical difference in the Foot and Ankle Outcome Questionnaire and Kitaoka Foot Scores despite similar bimodal distribution and clinical presentation to those observed by Ouzounian and Anderson.[14] Kopp and colleagues[33] analyzed the operative outcomes of 10 patients, 5 treated with primary repair and 5 with EHL or EDL tendon transfer. Surgical management resulted in a significant improvement in AOFAS scores and patient-reported pain, activity, and overall satisfaction. Dorsiflexion strength of the operative limb compared with the uninvolved extremity was significantly weaker; however, there was no difference between groups treated with repair versus tendon transfer. Because of small sample sizes, studies to date have been unable to provide any valid statistical means of comparing operative procedures, so this reflects an area of potential future studies within the literature.

With regard to time to treatment, Sammarco and colleagues[5] reviewed preoperative and postoperative assessments for 19 patients with early (<6 weeks from injury) and late anterior tibial tendon ruptures. They found significant improvements in AOFAS hindfoot scores, dorsiflexion strength, and gait pattern analysis for both early and late operative treatment. However, the sample size was too small to compare the means between early and late treatment or direct repair versus autograft reconstruction.

SUMMARY

Rupture of the TA tendon is a rare injury that has primarily been studied through case reports and low-volume case studies. Common mechanisms of injury include direct trauma, closed indirect trauma, an applied dorsiflexion force, or spontaneous rupture. The site of spontaneous rupture corresponds with an avascular zone beneath the inferior and superior extensor retinaculum. Patients typically present with signs and symptoms including anterior ankle pain, a palpable tendon defect, drop-foot gait, and decreased dorsiflexion strength. Most elderly, low-demand patients can be managed with nonoperative treatment with immobilization in an AFO with few functional limitations. Young, active, high-demand patients can be treated with a variety of surgical options, including primary repair, tendon transfer, and autograft or allograft reconstruction depending on the chronicity of the injury and size of the defect. Studies comparing nonoperative and surgical outcomes are limited with mixed results, but generally reflect the need to treat the bimodal distribution of patient cases accordingly. The most common residual deficit following operative management is decreased dorsiflexion strength compared with the nonoperative limb. Further studies are needed to evaluate the comparative efficacy of primary repair, tendon transfer, and autograft and allograft reconstruction.

REFERENCES

1. Anagnostakos K, Bachelier F, Furst OA, et al. Rupture of the anterior tibial tendon: three clinical cases, anatomical study, and literature review. Foot Ankle Int 2006; 27(5):330–9.

2. Coughlin M, Schon L. Chapter 24 disorder of tendons: anterior tibial tendon rupture. In: Mann's surgery of the foot and ankle. 9th edition. Philadelphia(PA): Saunders; 2014. p. 1197–209.

3. Petersen W, Stein V, Tillmann B. Blood supply of the tibialis anterior tendon. Arch Orthop Trauma Surg 1999;119(7–8):371–5.

4. Beischer AD, Beamond BM, Jowett AJ, et al. Distal tendinosis of the tibialis anterior tendon. Foot Ankle Int 2009;30(11):1053–9.

5. Sammarco VJ, Sammarco GJ, Henning C, et al. Surgical repair of acute and chronic tibialis anterior tendon ruptures. J Bone Joint Surg Am 2009;91(2): 325–32.

6. Grundy JR, O'Sullivan RM, Beischer AD. Operative management of distal tibialis anterior tendinopathy. Foot Ankle Int 2010;31(3):212–9.

7. Forst R, Forst J, Heller KD. Ipsilateral peroneus brevis tendon grafting in a complicated case of traumatic rupture of tibialis anterior tendon. Foot Ankle Int 1995; 16(7):440–4.

8. Dooley BJ, Kudelka P, Menelaus MB. Subcutaneous rupture of the tendon of tibialis anterior. J Bone Joint Surg Br 1980;62B(4):471–2.

9. Patten A, Pun WK. Spontaneous rupture of the tibialis anterior tendon: a case report and literature review. Foot Ankle Int 2000;21(8):697–700.

10. Otte S, Klinger HM, Lorenz F, et al. Operative treatment in case of a closed rupture of the anterior tibial tendon. Arch Orthop Trauma Surg 2002;122(3): 188–90.

11. Markarian GG, Kelikian AS, Brage M, et al. Anterior tibialis tendon ruptures: an outcome analysis of operative versus nonoperative treatment. Foot Ankle Int 1998;19(12):792–802.

12. Christman-Skieller C, Merz MK, Tansey JP. A systematic review of tibialis anterior tendon rupture treatments and outcomes. Am J Orthop (Belle Mead NJ) 2015; 44(4):E94–9.

13. Cohen DA, Gordon DH. The long-term effects of an untreated tibialis anterior tendon rupture. J Am Podiatr Med Assoc 1999;89(3):149–52.

14. Ouzounian TJ, Anderson R. Anterior tibial tendon rupture. Foot Ankle Int 1995; 16(7):406–10.

15. Ellington JK, McCormick J, Marion C, et al. Surgical outcome following tibialis anterior tendon repair. Foot Ankle Int 2010;31(5):412–7.

16. DiDomenico LA, Williams K, Petrolla AF. Spontaneous rupture of the anterior tibial tendon in a diabetic patient: results of operative treatment. J Foot Ankle Surg 2008;47(5):463–7.
17. Neumayer F, Djembi YR, Gerin A, et al. Closed rupture of the tibialis anterior tendon: a report of 2 cases. J Foot Ankle Surg 2009;48(4):457–61.
18. Goetz J, Beckmann J, Koeck F, et al. Gait analysis after tibialis anterior tendon rupture repair using Z-plasty. J Foot Ankle Surg 2013;52(5):598–601.
19. Sapkas GS, Tzoutzopoulos A, Tsoukas FC, et al. Spontaneous tibialis anterior tendon rupture: delayed repair with free-sliding tibialis anterior tendon graft. Am J Orthop (Belle Mead NJ) 2008;37(12):E213–6.
20. Wong MW. Traumatic tibialis anterior tendon rupture-delayed repair with free sliding tibialis anterior tendon graft. Injury 2004;35(9):940–4.
21. Kashyap S, Prince R. Spontaneous rupture of the tibialis anterior tendon. A case report. Clin Orthop Relat Res 1987;(216):159–61.
22. Velan GJ, Hendel D. Degenerative tear of the tibialis anterior tendon after cortico-steroid injection–augmentation with the extensor hallucis longus tendon, case report. Acta Orthop Scand 1997;68(3):308–9.
23. Kelikian A, Kelikian H. Tendon disruptions and dislocations of same tendons. In: Jahss MH, editor. Disorders of the foot and ankle. 1st edition. Philadelphia: WB Saunders; 1985. p. 782–5.
24. Pinzur MS, Kett N, Trilla M. Combined anterior/posterior tibial tendon transfer in post-traumatic peroneal palsy. Foot Ankle 1988;8:271–5.
25. Stavrou P, Symeonidis PD. Gracilis tendon graft for tibialis anterior tendon reconstruction: a report of two cases. Foot Ankle Int 2008;29(7):742–5.
26. Yamazaki S, Majima T, Yasui K, et al. Reconstruction of chronic anterior tibial tendon defect using hamstring tendon graft: a case report. Foot Ankle Int 2007;28(11):1190–3.
27. Yasui Y, Takao M, Miyamoto W, et al. Reconstruction using an autograft with near complete preservation of the extensor retinaculum for chronic tibialis anterior tendon disruption. Arch Orthop Trauma Surg 2013;133(12):1669–73.
28. Michels F, Van Der Bauwhede J, Oosterlinck D, et al. Minimally invasive repair of the tibialis anterior tendon using a semitendinosus autograft. Foot Ankle Int 2014; 35(3):264–71.
29. Huh J, Boyette DM, Parekh SG, et al. Allograft reconstruction of chronic tibialis anterior tendon ruptures. Foot Ankle Int 2015;36(10):1180–9.
30. Aderinto J, Gross A. Delayed repair of tibialis anterior tendon rupture with Achilles tendon allograft. J Foot Ankle Surg 2011;50(3):340–2.
31. Eckel TT, Nunley JA. Botox as an adjuvant to tendon transfer for foot drop. J Surg Orthop Adv 2013;22(3):233–6.
32. Gwynne-Jones D, Garneti N, Wyatt M. Closed tibialis anterior tendon rupture: a case series. Foot Ankle Int 2009;30(8):758–62.
33. Kopp FJ, Backus S, Deland JT. Anterior tibial tendon rupture: results of operative treatment. Foot Ankle Int 2007;28(10):1045–7.

Acute Peroneal Injury

James W. Brodsky, MD[a,b,c], Jacob R. Zide, MD[a,b],
Justin M. Kane, MD[a,b],*

KEYWORDS

- Lateral ankle injuries • Peroneal tendons • Peroneal tendon abnormality

KEY POINTS

- A high clinical suspicion and greater understanding of the anatomy and pathophysiology of lateral ankle injuries have enabled early diagnosis and treatment-improving outcomes of acute peroneal tendon tears.
- Multiple conditions can be the cause of lateral ankle pain attributed to the peroneal tendons: tenosynovitis, tendinosis, subluxation and dislocation, stenosing tenosynovitis, abnormality related to the os peroneum, as well as tears of the peroneal tendons.
- It is imperative for the clinician to maintain a high suspicion for peroneal tendon abnormality when evaluating patients with lateral ankle pain.

INTRODUCTION

Although once thought to be a rare cause of lateral-sided ankle pain, a better understanding of the anatomy, mechanisms of injury, and different abnormalities has led to peroneal tendon tears being recognized as an important cause of lateral ankle pain. When pain is located posterior to the lateral malleolus, there should be a high clinical suspicion for peroneal tendon injuries.

A myriad of conditions can be the cause of lateral ankle pain attributed to the peroneal tendons: tenosynovitis, tendinosis, subluxation and dislocation, stenosing tenosynovitis, abnormality related to the os peroneum, as well as tears of the peroneal tendons. With respect to peroneal tendon tears, they can be categorized as either acute tears or chronic. It is important to understand the temporal relationship that separates acute from chronic is not the time to presentation. In fact, acute peroneal tears can present in a delayed fashion and are often not appreciated when they happen. Rather, acute tears invariably occur after a traumatic injury, and it is their relationship to an injury that categorizes them as acute. Chronic tears tend to be attritional in nature and have an insidious and gradual onset of pain.

The authors have nothing to disclose.
[a] Foot and Ankle Surgery Division, Baylor University Medical Center, 3500 Gaston Avenue, Dallas, TX 75246, USA; [b] Texas A&M University Health Science Center, 3302 Gaston Avenue, Dallas, TX 75246, USA; [c] Department of Orthopaedic Surgery, UT Southwestern, 5323 Harry Hines Boulevard, Dallas, TX 75390, USA
* Corresponding author.
E-mail address: jkane.md@gmail.com

Foot Ankle Clin N Am 22 (2017) 833–841
http://dx.doi.org/10.1016/j.fcl.2017.07.013
foot.theclinics.com

It is imperative for the clinician to maintain a high suspicion for peroneal tendon abnormality when evaluating patients with lateral ankle pain. Coupled with an understanding of the anatomy, biomechanics, the spectrum of disease states of the tendons, and numerous treatment options, the clinician can make the appropriate treatment decisions to maximize the patient's chance at recovery and return to activity.

ANATOMY

The lateral compartment of the lower leg comprises the peroneus brevis and peroneus longus muscles and tendons. Both muscles receive their innervation from the superficial peroneal nerve. The peroneus brevis originates at the interior two-thirds of the lateral fibula. It courses directly behind the fibula with its musculotendinous junction at a variable location. Typically, the musculotendinous junction lies proximal to the superior retinaculum (SPR); however, anatomic variation often results in a low-lying muscle belly that extends within or distal to the level of the SPR. A low-lying muscle belly has been identified as a potential cause for inflammation of the peroneals at the level of the SPR as a result of the increased volume within the retrofibular space.[1,2] The tendinous portion of the peroneus brevis is an ovoid shape. The insertion of the peroneus brevis is on the lateral surface of the fifth metatarsal base at the styloid process.

The peroneus longus originates more proximally at the head of the fibula and upper one-half to two-thirds of the lateral fibular shaft and the lateral condyle of the tibia. The musculotendinous junction is proximal to that of the peroneus brevis, and the tendon tends to have a more circular morphology. The insertion of the peroneus longus is on the plantar lateral aspects of the medial cuneiform and first metatarsal base.

As the tendons of the peroneus brevis and longus course distally, they enter into the retromalleolar groove under the SPR. The peroneus brevis lies closer to the fibula and glides along the fibrocartilage lining of the retromalleolar groove. Edwards[3] described the morphology of the retromalleolar groove. In 178 specimens, 82% were concave, ranging from slight concavity to 3 mm depth; 11% of specimens had a flat retromalleolar groove, and 7% had a slightly convex morphology. In most patients, the sulcus of the retromalleolar groove was 6- to 7 mm wide. A 3- to 4-cm-long ring of fibrocartilaginous tissue courses along the retromalleolar groove, increasing the stability of the tendons.[4] Although it has long been postulated that a flat or convex peroneal groove would be associated with peroneal instability, Adachi and colleagues[5] studied retromalleolar morphology and concluded that no correlation between the shape of the retromalleolar groove and dislocation could be identified.

Numerous studies have identified the SPR as the primary restraint to peroneal instability.[4,6,7] Davis and colleagues[7] described the morphology of the SPR. A common origin was identified along the periosteum of the posterolateral ridge of the fibula. Variation existed in the width of the footprint of the origin. Five distinct insertions were described.

Both tendons share a common tendon sheath beginning approximately 2.5 to 3.5 cm proximal to the tip of the fibula until they reach the level of the peroneal tubercle. The 2 tendons then separate into individual tendon sheaths with the peroneus brevis above the peroneal tubercle and the peroneus longus below. The peroneus longus then courses plantar to the peroneus brevis and turns medially at the cuboid groove before reaching its insertion.

The os peroneum is a sesamoid bone in the peroneus longus just proximal to the cuboid groove. It has varying degrees of ossification and is reported to be present in up to 20% of patients in anatomic studies.[8] It is important to recognize the os peroneum as a potential pain generator. Fractures of the os peroneum are frequently painful, are often missed, and have a high correlation with peroneus longus tears.

The blood supply to both muscles arises from the peroneal artery. Petersen and colleagues[9] conducted a cadaveric study to better elucidate the blood supply to the tendons. The peroneus brevis has a single avascular zone near the distal tip of the fibula as the tendon makes its turn toward its insertion. Two avascular zones were identified in the peroneus longus: the first, as the tendon courses from the distal tip of the fibula to the peroneal tubercle; the second, as the tendon courses through the cuboid notch. This pattern of avascularity makes intuitive sense as it correlates to frequent areas of tendonopathy.

The peroneus quartus is an anatomic variant that is present in up to 21.7% of the population. It originates from the peroneus brevis muscle belly and inserts on the peroneal tubercle. It is postulated that the traction of the peroneus quartus can result in hypertrophy of the peroneal tubercle. The peroneus quartus tendon and hypertrophy of the peroneal tubercle can both lead to stenosing synovitis.[10]

BIOMECHANICS

Physiologic hindfoot valgus is essential for proper functioning of balance of the peroneal tendons. An excessively valgus hindfoot alignment may result in subfibular impingement and tendinosis as the tendons are compressed between the fibular tip and lateral calcaneus. A varus hindfoot alignment may put increased strain on the peroneal tendons predisposing to a spectrum of peroneal abnormality.

The peroneal tendons are the primary evertors of the foot. Sixty-three percent of eversion strength can be attributed to the peroneal tendons with the peroneus brevis responsible for 28% and the peroneus longus responsible for 35%.[11] They are the counterbalance to the tibialis posterior and anterior, respectively. In addition to everting the foot, they have a minor contribution to plantarflexion (4%) because they course posterior to the midaxis of the tibiotalar joint in the sagittal plane. They also play a vital role in the dynamic stability of the ankle.

Mann[12] described the peroneal tendons' function through the gait cycle. They are active during the stance phase of gait, initiating firing at 12% of the gait cycle. At midstance with the foot flat on the floor, the tendons fire eccentrically. At heel raise, they begin to contract concentrically. They become quiescent at 50% of the gait cycle just before toe off.

INCIDENCE AND CAUSE

Acute tears tend to be less common than chronic tears, and a high degree of clinical suspicion is needed for accurate diagnosis. Sammarco[13] noted that despite the acute onset of symptoms, after sustaining a traumatic inversion injury, only one patient was diagnosed within 2 weeks of the trauma. The average duration of symptoms persisted from 7 to 48 months before diagnosis. In 75% of patients who presented with acute peroneus longus tears, a concomitant peroneus brevis tear was identified. Arbab and colleagues[14] also noted the relative delay in diagnosis with acute peroneal tears. In their series, an accurate diagnosis was made approximately 11 months after the onset of symptoms. Again, all patients presented with acute onset of symptoms after sustaining a traumatic ankle injury: inversion injury. Additional studies identifying acute cases of peroneal tendon ruptures exist mostly in case report format. The overwhelming theme is that in cases of acute tendon rupture, an antecedent inversion-type ankle injury occurred, and the longus tendon was disproportionately affected.[15–17]

The overall incidence of acute and chronic peroneal tendon tears is recognized to be much more common than previously thought. In a cadaveric study, Sobel and colleagues[18] found a 37% (21/57) incidence of peroneus brevis tears. Most of these were found within the retrofibular groove. Given their location, they concluded that mechanical trauma was a likely cause of the tearing. In a study assessing the incidence of peroneus brevis abnormality in patients undergoing lateral ligament stabilization, Sammarco and DiRaimondo[19] noted that 23% (11/47) of patients had concomitant abnormality. DiGiovanni and colleagues[20] looked at the incidence of peroneal abnormality in patients treated surgically for chronic lateral ankle instability. Tenosynovitis was noted in 77% of patients; attenuation of the SPR was noted in 54% of patients, and peroneus brevis tears were noted in 25% of patients. A radiographic study conducted by O'Neil and colleagues[21] looked at 294 MRIs obtained where no hindfoot abnormality was suspected. Some evidence of peroneal abnormality was identified in 35% (103/294) despite a lack of symptoms or antecedent injury.

Several studies have investigated the actual incidence of tendon involvement when abnormality of the peroneal tendons is present. Dombek and colleagues[22] reported a rate of peroneus brevis tears in 88% of surgically treated patients for peroneal abnormality. Only 13% of patients had peroneus longus tears. Concomitant tears of both tendons have been reported in up to 38% of patients.[23]

Although most peroneus brevis tears occur in the retromalleolar groove, peroneus longus tears have 2 distinct patterns of tearing. Brandes and Smith[24] categorized peroneus longus tears by location. When tearing was noted to occur at the cuboid notch, 100% of them were complete tears. In patients with tears near the peroneal tubercle, 8/9 had a partial tear. The study additionally noted that there was a higher propensity for concomitant peroneus brevis tears when the peroneus tendon was affected at the cuboid notch. Thompson and Patterson[25] noted the markedly reduced frequency of peroneus longus tears in comparison with brevis tears. They usually occurred after a trauma or sports-related injury. The role of sports-related injuries in peroneus longus ruptures was further identified by Kilkelly and McHale.[26]

CLINICAL PRESENTATION

Making the diagnosis of an acute peroneal tendon tear is quite difficult. Invariably, the patient with the acute tear has sustained an inversion injury resulting in lateral-sided ankle or hindfoot swelling and pain. Thus, on initial presentation, differentiation of a peroneal tear from an ankle sprain can be a challenge. In this setting, there therefore must be a high clinical suspicion for peroneal abnormality given the myriad of other abnormalities that present as lateral-sided ankle pain. Studies have estimated a delay in diagnosis of peroneal tears ranging from 11 to 48 months with very few cases being diagnosed on initial presentation.[13,14] Although making the diagnosis of a peroneal tear acutely may not necessarily alter the acute treatment of the patient, it is important in patient guidance with regard to their rehabilitation potential and possible need for future surgical intervention.

Inspection of the affected extremity is the first step in making an accurate diagnosis. Standing examination is critical because hindfoot varus is thought to contribute to the incidence of peroneal tendon abnormality. In one study, 82% of patients with peroneus longus abnormality had a cavovarus alignment.[24] This was further expanded upon by Manoli and Graham.[27] In patients with peroneus brevis tears, retrofibular swelling is commonly encountered.[28] Redfern and Myerson[23] found that when swelling and pain occurs adjacent to the tip of the fibula, there is a high likelihood of peroneus brevis tears and both tendon involvement is possible. Swelling more distal at the base of the fifth metatarsal especially when it extends into the cuboid notch is more likely to signify a peroneus longus tear.[29]

In patients in which swelling is absent, pain with palpation at the retromalleolar groove as well as ankle instability can indicate split tearing of the peroneus brevis. Pain and instability may be the only presenting symptoms with an absence of swelling.[30,31]

Certain physical examination maneuvers may help identify peroneal tendon abnormality. Passive inversion and plantarflexion may reproduce pain. Resisted eversion and dorsiflexion of the ankle may result in pain and weakness. Often, when a peroneus longus tear is present, weakness and pain with first ray plantarflexion is present.

IMAGING

The first step in imaging of patients suspected of having peroneal tendon tears is to obtain a weight-bearing anteroposterior, oblique, and lateral radiograph of the foot and ankle. Plain films should be inspected for common fractures associated with inversion injuries, such as fractures of the malleoli, lateral talar process, anterior process of the calcaneus, and fifth metatarsal base. An avulsion from the lateral aspect of the distal fibula may be a fleck sign, indicative of rupture of the peroneal retinaculum.

Although the tendons themselves obviously cannot be seen on radiograph, certain radiographic findings can indicate a tendon rupture. Migration of the os peroneum or diastasis of a bipartite os peroneum has been described in several studies as a clear indicator of peroneus longus rupture.[26,32,33] Stockton and Brodsky[34] described radiographic evidence of a fracture or proximal migration of the os peroneum in 87.5% of surgically confirmed cases of peroneus longus ruptures. Although not a pathognomonic indicator of peroneus brevis tearing, fractures of the styloid process at the base of the fifth metatarsal have been associated with brevis tears.[35]

MRI is the ideal modality for evaluating soft tissue lesions. Acute peroneal tears will have increased signal intensity on T2-weighted imaging. Tearing of the peroneus brevis may appear as bisected, flattened, or C-shaped.[36] Khoury and colleagues[37] described peroneus longus tears as having a linear or round area of increased signal intensity within the tendon on T2 imaging. Stockton and Brodsky[34] described bony edema, visible fractures, and diastasis of the os peroneum as evidence of a peroneus longus tear. Unfortunately, although MRI is the ideal modality for evaluating soft tissue, there are difficulties when evaluating for peroneal tendon tears. Because of the course of the peroneal tendons, there is susceptibility to the so-called magic angle effect. The magic angle effect is a magnetic phenomenon that occurs when the tendon is oriented 55° to the axis of the magnetic field, and increased signal intensity as a result of the angular orientation can be seen and misdiagnosed as abnormality.[38] It has been suggested that an oblique orientation of the MRI beam at the midfoot may improve the accuracy in diagnosing peroneus longus tears[39] because this should mitigate the magic angle effect.

Stockton and Brodsky[34] described variable diagnostic accuracy with MRI compared with surgical exploration. They recommend using experienced radiologists who understand the abnormality being evaluated. Although Brandes and Smith[24] described MRI as overestimating the severity of peroneal tears, Redfern and Myerson[23] found that MRI may underestimate the extent of the abnormality, especially as it pertains to peroneus longus tears. Lamm and colleagues[40] reported an 83% sensitivity and 75% specificity compared with intraoperative findings for brevis tears. They described the findings associated with brevis tears as flattening in MRIs obtained with the patient in both plantarflexion and dorsiflexion. Park and colleagues[41] compared 97 MRIs to surgical results and concluded that MRI was specific for diagnosing peroneal tendon disorders but not sensitive. Giza and colleagues[42] correlated clinical examination with MRI findings and found a positive predictive value of MRI to be only 48% with a high rate of incidental findings. This was further confirmed by O'Neil and colleagues,[21] who found incidental finding suggestive of peroneal tendon abnormality in 35% of asymptomatic patients. These variations in MRI findings correlating to surgical findings make it difficult to ascertain the true utility of MRI.

In the hands of an experienced diagnostician, ultrasound is an efficacious modality. It is inexpensive and radiation free and can be used for both diagnosis and treatment. Grant and colleagues[13] found ultrasound to be 100% sensitive and 85% specific for diagnosing peroneal tendon tears. Molini and Bianchi[44] found ultrasound to be a noninvasive, accurate, low-morbidity dynamic examination in which there was no radiation exposure. In a study looking at the accuracy of peroneal tendon sheath injection, Muir and colleagues[45] found ultrasound to be 100% accurate for intrasheath injection.

Treatment

Because a paucity of literature exists regarding an optimal treatment algorithm, it follows that a vast array of treatment protocols exists among practitioners when treating peroneal tendon tears. Grice and colleagues[46] queried foot and ankle surgeons on their management of acute peroneal tendon tears. There were marked differences in treatment protocols as well as operative techniques. Nonoperative treatment for greater than 1 year was undertaken by 22% of surgeons, whereas 33% of surgeons forwent any nonoperative interventions. When operative intervention was undertaken, 88% of surgeons tubularized tendons after repair; 33% excised redundant tissue, and 22% removed the peroneal tubercle if it was hypertrophied. A variety of suture materials were used, and postoperative protocols varied widely. This study was echoed by that of Sammarco.[13] In his case series, there was marked variability in the treatment of acute tears. Selmani and colleagues[47] reported poor evidence for type of repair for peroneal tendon tears.

Krause and Brodsky[28] proposed a treatment algorithm based on the amount of viable tendon remaining in cross-sectional diameter. They concluded that the treatment of peroneus brevis tears was primarily operative. For tendons with less than 50% involvement, excision and tubularization was the preferred treatment. For tendons with greater than 50% involvement, excision of the diseased tendon with tenodesis was the preferred treatment.

Redfern and Myerson[23] proposed an alternative treatment algorithm. They categorized tears into 3 patterns. Type I tears were where both tendons were intact and functioning. The torn portion of the tendon could be excised and tubularized. Type II tears were where one tendon was torn and irreparable with the other was still functional. In these cases, excision of the irreparable part of the tendon with tenodesis should be performed. Type III tears were where neither tendon was functional. In these cases, a tendon transfer was the optimal treatment.[23]

Outcomes

Although the current body of literature is lacking of high-quality evidence supporting the outcomes for the surgical treatment of peroneal tears, more recent reviews suggest that many patients do well with the ability to return to their preinjury activities.

Most studies report relatively positive outcomes with surgically treated peroneal tears. It is paramount to accurately diagnose patients with peroneal tendon tears in order to ensure successful and predictable outcomes.[14] Krause and Brodsky[28] reported a 95% satisfaction rate with surgical treatment of peroneal tendon tears with a mean postoperative American Orthopaedic Foot and Ankle Society (AOFAS) score of 85 (54–100).[28] In the study conducted by Redfern and Myerson,[23] these results were echoed. There was mean postoperative AOFAS score of 82 with 91% of patients achieving normal or moderate peroneal strength. It was noted that peroneus brevis tears fared better surgically than longus tears. Another study reported a mean postoperative AOFAS score of 91 with 87% of patients returning to sporting activity in an average of 3.5 months.[48] Demetracopoulos and colleagues[49] reported on the long-term results of primary repair of peroneal tendon tears. A statistically significant reduction in visual analogue score from 39 to 10 ($P<.001$) was detected with a statistically significant increase in lower extremity function score from 45 to 71 ($P<.001$). All but one patient was able to make a full return to sports-related activity.[49] In a retrospective review of surgically treated peroneal tendon tears, Dombek and colleagues[22] reported 98% of patients had no limitations at final follow-up without any pain. They did note a minor complication rate of 20%, which was defined as transient symptoms. Their incidence of major complications, which entailed persistent symptoms or a need for further surgery, was noted to be 10%. In a study involving the surgical treatment of all peroneal abnormalities excluding subluxations, it was reported that the average time to return to work was 2.5 months with an average time to return to sporting activity 8.5 months. All but one patient was either satisfied or very satisfied with their procedure (94.1%).[50]

SUMMARY

Although once thought to be uncommon, a high clinical suspicion and greater understanding of the anatomy and pathophysiology of lateral ankle injuries have enabled early diagnosis and treatment improving outcomes of acute peroneal tendon tears.

REFERENCES

1. Roster B, Michelier P, Giza E. Peroneal tendon disorders. Clin Sports Med 2015; 34(4):525–641.
2. Kelikian AS. Sarrafians anatomy of the foot and ankle: descriptive, topographic, functional. 3rd edition. Philadelphia: J.B. Lippincott; 2011.
3. Edwards ME. Relations of peroneal tendons to fibula, calcaneus, and cuboideum. Am J Anat 1928;42:213–53.
4. Eckert WR, Davis EA Jr. Acute rupture of the peroneal retinaculum. J Bone Joint Surg 1976;58A:670–3.
5. Adachi N, Fukuhara K, Kobyashi T, et al. Morphologic variations of the fibular malleolar groove with recurrent dislocation of the peroneal tendons. Foot Ankle Int 2009;30(6):540–4.
6. Niemi WJ, Savidakis J Jr, DeJesus JM. Peroneal subluxation: a comprehensive review of the literature with case presentations. J Foot Ankle Surg 1997;36:141–5.
7. Davis WH, Sobel M, Deland J, et al. The superior peroneal retinaculum: an anatomic study. Foot Ankle Int 1994;15:271–5.
8. Sobel M, Pavlov H, Geppert MJ, et al. Painful os peroneum, syndrome: a spectrum of conditions responsible for plantar lateral foot pain. Foot Ankle Int 1994; 15(3):112–24.
9. Petersen W, Bobka T, Stein V, et al. Blood supply of the peroneal tendons. Injection and immunohistochemical studies of cadaver tendons. Acta Orthop Scand 2000;71:168–74.

10. Sobel M, Levy ME, Bohne WH. Congenital variations of the peroneus quartus muscle: an anatomic study. Foot Ankle Int 1990;11:81–9.
11. Clark HD, Kitaoka HB, Ehman RL. Peroneal tendon injuries. Foot Ankle Int 1998; 19(5):280–8.
12. Mann RA. Overview of the foot and ankle biomechanics. Disorders of the foot and ankle: medical and surgical management. 2nd edition. Philadelphia: WB Saunders; 1991.
13. Sammarco GJ. Peroneus longus tendon tears: acute and chronic. Foot Ankle Int 1995;16(5):245–53.
14. Arbab D, Tingart M, Frank D, et al. Treatment of isolated peroneus longus tears and a review of the literature. Foot Ankle Spec 2014;7(2):113–8.
15. Abraham E, Stirnaman JE. Neglected rupture of the peroneal tendons causing recurrent sprains of the ankle. Case report. J Bone Joint Surg Am 1979;61(8). 1247–8.
16. Davies JA. Peroneal compartment syndrome secondary to rupture of the peroneus longus. A case report. J Bone Joint Surg Am 1979;61(5):783–4.
17. Evans JD. Subcutaneous rupture of the tendon of peroneus longus. Report of a case. J Bone Joint Surg Br 1966;48(3):507–9.
18. Sobel M, DiCarlo EF, Bohne WH, et al. Longitudinal splitting of the peroneus brevis tendon: an anatomic and histologic study of cadaveric material. Foot Ankle 1991;12(3):165–70.
19. Sammarco GJ, DiRaimondo CV. Chronic peroneus brevis tendon lesions. Foot Ankle 1989;9(4):163–70.
20. DiGiovanni BF, Fraga CJ, Cohen BE, et al. Associated injuries found in chronic lateral ankle instability. Foot Ankle Int 2000;21(1):809–15.
21. O'Neil JT, Pedowitz DI, Kerbel YE, et al. Peroneal tendon abnormalities on routine magnetic resonance imaging of the foot and ankle. Foot Ankle Int 2016;37(7): 743–7.
22. Dombek MF, Lamm BM, Saltrick K, et al. Peroneal tendon tears: a retrospective review. J Foot Ankle Surg 2003;42:250–8.
23. Redfern D, Myerson M. The management of concomitant tears of the peroneus longus and brevis tendons. Foot Ankle Int 2004;25:695–707.
24. Brandes CB, Smith RW. Characterization of patients with primary longus tendinopathy: a review of twenty-two cases. Foot Ankle Int 2000;21(6):462–8.
25. Thompson FM, Patterson AH. Rupture of the peroneus longus tendon. Report of three cases. J Bone Joint Surg Am 1989;71(2):293–5.
26. Kilkelly FX, McHale KAS. Acute rupture of the peroneal longus tendon in a runner: a case report and review of the literature. Foot Ankle Int 1994;15:567–9.
27. Manoli A 2nd, Graham B. The subtle cavus foot, "the underpronator". Foot Ankle Int 2005;26(3):256–63.
28. Krause JO, Brodsky JW. Peroneus brevis tendon tears: pathophysiology, surgical reconstruction, and clinical results. Foot Ankle Int 1998;19(5):271–9.
29. Slater HK. Acute peroneal tendon tears. Foot Ankle Clin 2007;12(4):659–74.
30. Bonnin M, Tavernier T, Bouysset M. Split lesions of the peroneus brevis tendon in chronic ankle laxity. Am J Sports Med 1997;25(5):699–703.
31. Sobel M, Geppert MJ, Olson EJ, et al. The dynamics of peroneus brevis tendon splits: a proposed mechanism, technique of diagnosis, and classification of injury. Foot Ankle 1992;13:413–22.
32. Bianchi S, Abdelwahab IF, Tegaldo G. Fracture and posterior dislocation of the os peroneum associated with rupture of the peroneus longus tendon. Can Assoc Radiol J 1991;42(5):340–4.

33. Tehranadeh J, Stoll DA, Gabriele OM. Case report 271. Posterior migration of the os peroneum of the left foot, indicating a tear of the peroneal tendon. Skeletal Radiol 1984;12(1):44–7.
34. Stockton KG, Brodsky JW. Peroneus longus tears associated with pathology of the os peroneum. Foot Ankle Int 2014;35(4):346–52.
35. Brigido MK, Fessell DP, Jacobson JA, et al. Radiography and US of os peroneum fractures and associated peroneal tendon injuries: initial experience. Radiology 2005;237:235–41.
36. Major NM, Helms CA, Fritz RC, et al. The MR imaging appearance of longitudinal split tears of the peroneus brevis tendon. Foot Ankle Int 2000;21:514–9.
37. Khoury NJ, el-Khoury GY, Saltzman CL, et al. Peroneus longus and brevis tendon tears: MR imaging evaluation. Radiology 1996;200:833–41.
38. Erickson SJ, Prost RW, Timins ME. The "magic angle" effect: background physics and clinical relevance. Radiology 1993;188(1):23–5.
39. Rademaker J, Rosenberg ZS, Delfaut EM, et al. Tears of the peroneus longus tendon: MR imaging features in nine patients. Radiology 2000;214:700–4.
40. Lamm BM, Myers DT, Dombek M, et al. Magnetic resonance imaging and surgical correlation of peroneus brevis tears. J Foot Ankle Surg 2004;43:30–6.
41. Park HJ, Lee SY, Park NH, et al. Accuracy of MR findings in characterizing peroneal tendon disorders in comparison with surgery. Acta Radiol 2012;53:795–801.
42. Giza E, Mak W, Wong SE, et al. A clinical and radiological study of peroneal tendon pathology. Foot Ankle Spec 2013;6(6):417–21.
43. Grant TH, Kelikian AS, Jereb SE, et al. Ultrasound diagnosis of peroneal tendon tears. A surgical correlation. J Bone Joint Surg Am 2005;87:1788–94.
44. Molini L, Bianchi S. US in peroneal tendon tear. J Ultrasound 2014;17(2):125–34.
45. Muir JJ, Curtiss HM, Hollman J, et al. The accuracy of ultrasound-guided and palpation-guided peroneal tendon sheath injections. Am J Phys Med Rehabil 2011;90(7):564–71.
46. Grice J, Watura C, Elliot R. Audit of foot and ankle surgeons' management of acute peroneal tendon tears and review of management protocols. Foot (Edinb) 2016;26:1–3.
47. Selmani E, Gjata V, Gjika E. Current concepts review: peroneal tendon disorders. Foot Ankle Int 2006;27(3):221–8.
48. Saxena A, Cassidy A. Peroneal tendon injuries: an evaluation of 49 tears in 41 patients. J Foot Ankle Surg 2003;42:215–20.
49. Demetracopoulos CA, Vineyard JC, Kiesau CD, et al. Long-term results of debridement and primary repair of peroneal tendon tears. Foot Ankle Int 2014;35(3):252–7.
50. Grasset W, Mercier N, Chaussard C, et al. The surgical treatment of peroneal tendinopathy (excluding subluxations): a series of 17 patients. J Foot Ankle Surg 2012;51(1):13–9.

Chronic Rupture of the Peroneal Tendons

Kamran S. Hamid, MD, MPH[a],*, Annunziato Amendola, MD[b]

KEYWORDS

- Chronic rupture • Peroneal tendons • Surgical solutions

KEY POINTS

- Chronic rupture of the peroneal tendons can be a functionally limiting condition with a multitude of causes.
- Conservative and operative interventions are heterogenous and tailored to the functional demands of the patient.
- Surgical plans are based on muscle viability, patient preference, and surgeon expertise.
- Clinical outcomes evidence remains limited in this domain, and further well-designed studies are warranted to guide treatment.

INTRODUCTION

Chronic rupture of the peroneal tendons may be the result of a neglected injury, chronic inflammatory changes, or the sequela of longstanding tension or friction that subjects the peroneal tendons to excessive stress leading to tendinopathy and subsequent discontinuity.[1–3] Abnormality can occur at the peroneus longus, peroneus brevis, or both tendons. A meticulous history, thorough physical examination, and appropriate diagnostic testing are imperative to identify the cause of this condition. Conservative and operative interventions are heterogenous and tailored to the functional demands of the patient.

Clinical Presentation

Patients with chronic ruptures of the peroneal tendons present with difficulty in hindfoot eversion, pain, swelling, and functional instability. Plantarflexion of the first ray or pivoting or ankle and dorsiflexion at the ankle may prove difficult as well. Pain along the plantar aspect of the foot may indicate peroneus longus rupture or tendinopathy. History taking should attempt to elicit possible pathologic causes, including history of fluoroquinolone usage, steroid injection, prior trauma, infection, antecedent pain and swelling, chronic dislocating tendons, wearing out of lateral border of shoes due to

The authors have nothing to disclose.
[a] Rush University Medical Center, 1611 West Harrison Street, Chicago, Illinois 60612, USA;
[b] Duke University Medical Center, 4709 Creekstone Dr, Durham, NC 27703, USA
* Corresponding author.
E-mail address: kamranhamid@gmail.com

foot position, and previous surgery.[2] Chronicity of symptoms is important to ascertain as prolonged disuse of lateral compartment musculature may lead to fatty atrophy and less utility of operative tendon salvage. History taking may have sensitivity but lacks specificity because there is a great amount of overlap with chronic peroneal tendinopathy without rupture. Severity of weakness is the most notable distinguishing factor, although this may be confounded by pain.

Physical examination should begin with visual assessment of lower extremity alignment. Visual assessment requires observing the patient preferably in shorts with knees visible. Varus tensioning is commonly the underlying factor and may be secondary to ankle or subtalar malalignment, supramalleolar deformity, or varus angulation at the lovol of tho knoo. Tcndornoss and edema may be noted over the trajectory of the peroneals. In addition to standard strength testing, special attention should be paid to discern weakness in resisted ankle eversion and resisted first ray plantarflexion as compared with the contralateral limb. During resisted strength testing, the peroneals should be palpated for continuity. Single-leg balance and heel raise often prove painful and challenging. The patient may concomitantly have abnormality of the lateral ankle ligamentous complex with generalized instability in this region.

Diagnostic Imaging

Plain film assessment should be undertaken to identify any confounding abnormalities, such as arthritic disease, fracture, or nonunion. A lateral radiograph can prove valuable for identifying a proximally migrated os peroneum in the case of peroneus longus rupture or os peroneum fracture.[4] In addition to foot films, ankle radiographs and hindfoot alignment films are necessary to identify malalignment in the supramalleolar, ankle, or subtalar locations. Similarly, knee radiographs may be indicated when knee malalignment is suspected. MRI has limitations in peroneal tendon assessment because the tendons have a curvilinear course at the level of the distal fibula, subjecting them to magic angle phenomenon, which can belie the true integrity of these tendons.[5] With advanced disease, MRI will be useful to demonstrate the extent of abnormality. There may be a role for MRI in plantarflexion to mitigate the effect of this phenomenon and lessen artifact. The authors advocate for proximal extension of the MRI beyond the ankle so as to identify any fatty infiltration of the peroneal muscle belies in cases of suspected chronic rupture. Ultrasound is a powerful tool for assessment of the peroneal tendons, although its utility is correlated with operator skill and familiarity.[6]

TREATMENT OPTIONS
Conservative Management

Treatment plans should be decided upon after engaging in the shared decision-making process with the patient and germane family members. Functional demands, pain level, and the patient's risks of surgery should all be considered. Nonoperative management may have a limited role in true chronic peroneal rupture but can be indicated in the appropriate patient. Patients with lower functional demands and higher relative risk of surgical complications may be candidates for a period of immobilization followed by physical therapy and bracing.[1] If flexible heel varus exists secondary to a dropped first ray, then custom orthoses with lateral forefoot posting to maintain the heel in neutral may prove helpful.

Two-Cable Surgical Solutions

In cases with limited muscular fatty infiltration and preserved motor function, the impetus to proceed with surgery is heightened in order to optimize outcomes.

Tenodesis between the peroneals is a time-tested procedure with satisfactory results[7]; however, there has been a contemporary push toward preservation of native kinematics by conserving the independence of both peroneus longus and brevis cables. Multiple techniques have been described to facilitate this end.

The use of a Hunter rod was originally described in 1971 for 2-stage reconstruction of tendons in the hand.[8] A similar method in the ankle uses the temporary Hunter rod implant to generate a healthy peroneal tendon sheath to host a flexor hallucis longus (FHL) tendon transfer. This method of creating a healthy biologic membrane using a foreign body is akin to the Masquelet technique espoused by traumatologists for 2-stage segmental bone loss management.[9] Because of the rarity of this abnormality, clinical outcomes research is limited and often relegated to case series. Wapner and colleagues[10] demonstrated good results with the 2-stage reconstruction in 6 out of 7 patients undergoing the procedure at an average of 8.5-years follow-up.

Although the aforementioned technique avoids tenodesis, FHL transfer limits a true attempt at preserving natural kinematics. Spanning the gap between tendon ends after debridement may be conducted in multiple ways. Rapley and colleagues[11] used an acellular dermal matrix to span the tendinous gap and found improvement in American Orthopaedic Foot & Ankle Society score, pain, and function in a cohort of 7 patients requiring a "gap jump." Per the investigators, eversion strength improved to within half a motor grade as compared with the contralateral limb on average. Four additional patients underwent debridement with acellular dermal matrix wrapped as an augment but did not have true chronic rupture gap abnormality. Follow-up averaged 16.9 months in this series; thus long-term functionality is uncertain.

Mook and colleagues[12] evaluated 14 patients with peroneus longus and tendon ruptures requiring reconstruction of both. Mean follow-up was similar to Rapley and colleagues[11] at 17 months. The average length of the intercalary segment reconstructed was 10.8 cm, and average postoperative visual analogue score decreased to 1.0. Average postoperative eversion strength as categorized by the Medical Research Council grading scale improved to 4.8 ± 0.5 ($P = .001$). The average Short Form-12 score improved to 48.8 ± 7.8 ($P = .02$). Four patients experienced sural nerve sensory numbness, and 2 of these were transient. There were no postoperative wound healing complications, infections, tendon reruptures, or reoperations. No allograft-associated complications were identified. All 14 patients returned to their preinjury activity levels. A similar technique with autologous free graft from the peroneus brevis to longus with plantaris augment has been described in a case report[13].

One-Cable Surgical Solutions

In instances of chronic rupture-induced muscular atrophy and fatty degeneration, preservation of both peroneus longus and brevis function may not be feasible, and tenodesis is preferred. Patient and surgeon preference may also be indications for tenodesis because it is a time-tested procedure. Tenodesis involves debridement of nonviable tissue and anastomosis of the discontinuous tendon to the healthy tendon. Although tenodesis is a commonly used procedure in the setting of chronic peroneal rupture, this technique is extrapolated from its usage for large peroneal tears.[14,15] The external validity of these studies as related to this distinct abnormality is unvalidated.

There are no case-control or cohort studies comparing allograft reconstruction to tenodesis in the literature at this time. Pellegrini and colleagues[16] demonstrated in a cadaveric model that allograft reconstruction of a peroneus brevis tendon restored distal tension when the peroneal tendons and their antagonists were loaded to 50% and 100% of physiologic load. In contradistinction, tenodesis of the brevis to the peroneus longus tendon did not effectively restore peroneus brevis tension under comparable tested conditions. The investigators hypothesized that tenodesis may thus result in an imbalanced foot, although this assertion has not been clinically verified. Tenodesis takedown and conversion to dual allograft reconstructed peroneals have been promoted as a technique but without objective outcome measures as evidence.[17]

CLINICAL CASE

A 63-year-old male surgeon presented with several months of left posterolateral ankle pain and swelling that had worsened recently and is now functionally limiting in eversion and dorsiflexion. He denies fluoroquinolones, steroid usage, or an injury mecha nism. Upon examination in the clinic, the patient has genu varum bilaterally that is more pronounced on the left and reflected in standing leg length radiographs (**Fig. 1**). The patient has 1/5 strength in eversion, 3/5 strength in dorsiflexion, inability to plantarflex the first ray, and tenderness over the peroneals. MRI demonstrated chronic rupture abnormality of the peroneus longus tendon, attrition of the peroneus brevis, with peroneal sheath edema (**Fig. 2**).

After exhausting conservative treatment modalities, the patient opted for surgical intervention in a staged manner to correct his mechanical alignment and address his rupture abnormality. After high tibial osteotomy to correct genu varum, the patient underwent peroneal exploration. Intraoperatively, a ruptured and edematous peroneus longus tendon was identified. There was significant attrition of the peroneus brevis (**Fig. 3**). The nonviable portion of the ruptured ends was debrided, leaving an 8-cm gap distance (**Fig. 4**). A tibialis anterior allograft was used to bridge the gap in some

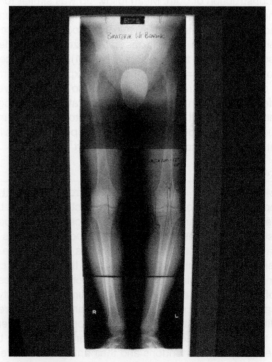

Fig. 1. Standing leg length films demonstrate pronounced left lower extremity genu varum and deviation from the mechanical axis.

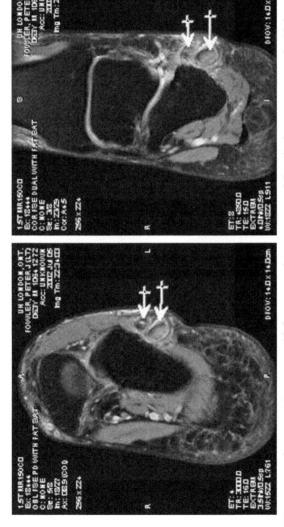

Fig. 2. Coronal MRI sequences demonstrating ruptured left peroneus longus rupture (*A*) and edema as compared with brevis (*B*). *Arrows* point to the diseased peroneus longus and brevis tendons.

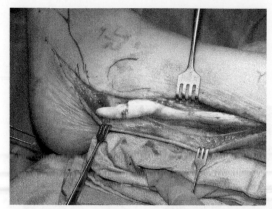

Fig. 3. Edematous remnant of chronic ruptured peroneus longus.

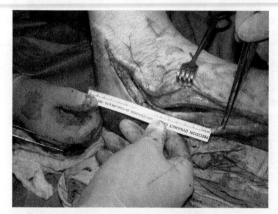

Fig. 4. Peroneus longus debrided and left with 8-cm gap distance.

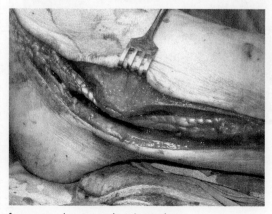

Fig. 5. Tenodesis of peroneus longus to brevis tendon.

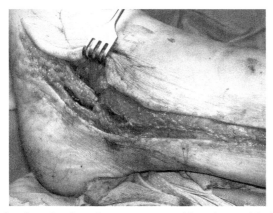

Fig. 6. Repair of sheath and retinaculum to prevent subluxation and facilitate gliding.

tension, and the longus tendon and graft were tenodesed to the brevis tendon (**Fig. 5**). The peroneal sheath and retinacular layers were tightly repaired to facilitate gliding and prevent subluxation or dislocation (**Fig. 6**). At long-term follow-up, the patient's pain and function both improved to allow excellent function as a surgeon and in his recreational life.

SUMMARY

Chronic rupture of the peroneal tendons can be a functionally limiting condition with a multitude of causes. Conservative and operative interventions are heterogenous and tailored to the functional demands of the patient. Surgical plans are based on muscle viability, patient preference, and surgeon expertise. Clinical outcomes evidence remains limited in this domain, and further well-designed studies are warranted to guide treatment.

REFERENCES

1. Dombek MF, Lamm BM, Saltrick K, et al. Peroneal tendon tears: a retrospective review. J Foot Ankle Surg 2003;42:250–8.
2. Krause JO, Brodsky JW. Peroneus brevis tendon tears: pathophysiology, surgical reconstruction, and clinical results. Foot Ankle Int 1998;19:271–9.
3. Redfern D, Myerson M. The management of concomitant tears of the peroneus longus and brevis tendons. Foot Ankle Int 2004;25:695–707.
4. Stockton KG, Brodsky JW. Peroneus longus tears associated with pathology of the os peroneum. Foot Ankle Int 2014;35:346–52.
5. Cerrato RA, Myerson MS. Peroneal tendon tears, surgical management and its complications. Foot Ankle Clin 2009;14:299–312.
6. Bruin DB, von Piekartz H. Musculoskeletal management of a patient with a history of chronic ankle sprains: identifying rupture of peroneal brevis and peroneal longus with diagnostic ultrasonography. J Chiropr Med 2014;13:203–9.
7. Stamatis ED, Karaoglanis GC. Salvage options for peroneal tendon ruptures. Foot Ankle Clin 2014;19(1):87–95.
8. Hunter JM, Salisbury RE. Flexor-tendon reconstruction in severely damaged hands. A two-stage procedure using a silicone-Dacron reinforced gliding prosthesis prior to tendon grafting. J Bone Joint Surg Am 1971;53:829–58.

9. Masquelet AC, Fitoussi F, Begue T, et al. Reconstruction of the long bones by the induced membrane and spongy autograft. Ann Chir Plast Esthet 2000;45:346–53 [in French].

10. Wapner KL, Taras JS, Lin SS, et al. Staged reconstruction for chronic rupture of both peroneal tendons using Hunter rod and flexor hallucis longus tendon transfer: a long-term followup study. Foot Ankle Int 2006;27:591–7.

11. Rapley JH, Crates J, Barber A. Mid-substance peroneal tendon defects augmented with an acellular dermal matrix allograft. Foot Ankle Int 2010;31: 136–40.

12. Mook WR, Parekh SG, Nunley JA. Allograft reconstruction of peroneal tendons: operative technique and clinical outcomes. Foot Ankle Int 2013;34:1212–20.

13. Mac M, Rodriguez A, Partoune E. Traumatic ruptures of the peroneal tendons treated by free autologous tendon graft. Acta Orthop Belg 1998;64:409–12 [in French].

14. Squires N, Myerson MS, Gamba C. Surgical treatment of peroneal tendon tears. Foot Ankle Clin 2007;12:675–95, vii.

15. Steginsky B, Riley A, Lucas DE, et al. Patient-reported outcomes and return to activity after peroneus brevis repair. Foot Ankle Int 2016;37:178–85.

16. Pellegrini MJ, Glisson RR, Matsumoto T, et al. Effectiveness of allograft reconstruction vs tenodesis for irreparable peroneus brevis tears: a cadaveric model. Foot Ankle Int 2016;37:803–8.

17. Pellegrini MJ, Adams SB, Parekh SG. Reversal of peroneal tenodesis with allograft reconstruction of the peroneus brevis and longus: case report and surgical technique. Foot Ankle Spec 2014;7:327–31.

UNITED STATES POSTAL SERVICE ®

Statement of Ownership, Management, and Circulation
(All Periodicals Publications Except Requester Publications)

1. Publication Title	2. Publication Number	3. Filing Date
FOOT AND ANKLE CLINICS OF NORTH AMERICA	016 – 368	9/18/2017

4. Issue Frequency	5. Number of Issues Published Annually	6. Annual Subscription Price
MAR, JUN, SEP, DEC	4	$320.00

7. Complete Mailing Address of Known Office of Publication (Not printer) (Street, city, county, state, and ZIP+4®)

ELSEVIER INC.
230 Park Avenue, Suite 800
New York, NY 10169

Contact Person
STEPHEN R. BUSHING

Telephone (Include area code)
215-239-3688

8. Complete Mailing Address of Headquarters or General Business Office of Publisher (Not printer)

ELSEVIER INC.
230 Park Avenue, Suite 800
New York, NY 10169

9. Full Names and Complete Mailing Addresses of Publisher, Editor, and Managing Editor (Do not leave blank)

Publisher (Name and complete mailing address)

ADRIANNE BRIGIDO, ELSEVIER INC.
1600 JOHN F KENNEDY BLVD. SUITE 1800
PHILADELPHIA, PA 19103-2899

Editor (Name and complete mailing address)

LAUREN BOYLE, ELSEVIER INC.
1600 JOHN F KENNEDY BLVD. SUITE 1800
PHILADELPHIA, PA 19103-2899

Managing Editor (Name and complete mailing address)

PATRICK MANLEY, ELSEVIER INC.
1600 JOHN F KENNEDY BLVD. SUITE 1800
PHILADELPHIA, PA 19103-2899

10. Owner (Do not leave blank. If the publication is owned by a corporation, give the name and address of the corporation immediately followed by the names and addresses of all stockholders owning or holding 1 percent or more of the total amount of stock. If not owned by a corporation, give the names and addresses of the individual owners. If owned by a partnership or other unincorporated firm, give its name and address as well as those of each individual owner. If the publication is published by a nonprofit organization, give its name and address.)

Full Name	Complete Mailing Address
WHOLLY OWNED SUBSIDIARY OF REED/ELSEVIER, US HOLDINGS	1600 JOHN F KENNEDY BLVD. SUITE 1800 PHILADELPHIA, PA 19103-2899

11. Known Bondholders, Mortgagees, and Other Security Holders Owning or Holding 1 Percent or More of Total Amount of Bonds, Mortgages, or Other Securities. If none, check box ☐ None

Full Name	Complete Mailing Address
N/A	

12. Tax Status (For completion by nonprofit organizations authorized to mail at nonprofit rates) (Check one)
The purpose, function, and nonprofit status of this organization and the exempt status for federal income tax purposes:
☒ Has Not Changed During Preceding 12 Months
☐ Has Changed During Preceding 12 Months (Publisher must submit explanation of change with this statement)

13. Publication Title	14. Issue Date for Circulation Data Below
FOOT AND ANKLE CLINICS OF NORTH AMERICA	JUNE 2017

15. Extent and Nature of Circulation			Average No. Copies Each Issue During Preceding 12 Months	No. Copies of Single Issue Published Nearest to Filing Date
a. Total Number of Copies (Net press run)			456	373
b. Paid Circulation (By Mail and Outside the Mail)	(1)	Mailed Outside-County Paid Subscriptions Stated on PS Form 3541 (Include paid distribution above nominal rate, advertiser's proof copies, and exchange copies)	281	243
	(2)	Mailed In-County Paid Subscriptions Stated on PS Form 3541 (Include paid distribution above nominal rate, advertiser's proof copies, and exchange copies)	0	0
	(3)	Paid Distribution Outside the Mails Including Sales Through Dealers and Carriers, Street Vendors, Counter Sales, and Other Paid Distribution Outside USPS®	112	99
	(4)	Paid Distribution by Other Classes of Mail Through the USPS (e.g. First-Class Mail®)	0	0
c. Total Paid Distribution (Sum of 15b (1), (2), (3), and (4))		▶	393	342
d. Free or Nominal Rate Distribution (By Mail and Outside the Mail)	(1)	Free or Nominal Rate Outside-County Copies included on PS Form 3541	29	31
	(2)	Free or Nominal Rate In-County Copies Included on PS Form 3541	0	0
	(3)	Free or Nominal Rate Copies Mailed at Other Classes Through the USPS (e.g. First-Class Mail)	0	0
	(4)	Free or Nominal Rate Distribution Outside the Mail (Carriers or other means)	0	0
e. Total Free or Nominal Rate Distribution (Sum of 15d (1), (2), (3) and (4))		▶	29	31
f. Total Distribution (Sum of 15c and 15e)		▶	422	373
g. Copies not Distributed (See Instructions to Publishers #4 (page #3))		▶	34	0
h. Total (Sum of 15f and g)		▶	456	373
i. Percent Paid (15c divided by 15f times 100)			93.13%	91.69%

* If you are claiming electronic copies, go to line 16 on page 3. If you are not claiming electronic copies, skip to line 17 on page 3.

16. Electronic Copy Circulation		Average No. Copies Each Issue During Preceding 12 Months	No. Copies of Single Issue Published Nearest to Filing Date
a. Paid Electronic Copies	▶	0	0
b. Total Paid Print Copies (Line 15c) + Paid Electronic Copies (Line 16a)	▶	393	342
c. Total Print Distribution (Line 15f) + Paid Electronic Copies (Line 16a)	▶	422	373
d. Percent Paid (Both Print & Electronic Copies) (16b divided by 16c × 100)	▶	93.13%	91.69%

☒ I certify that 50% of all my distributed copies (electronic and print) are paid above a nominal price.

17. Publication of Statement of Ownership

☒ If the publication is a general publication, publication of this statement is required. Will be printed ☐ Publication not required.
in the DECEMBER 2017 issue of this publication.

18. Signature and Title of Editor, Publisher, Business Manager, or Owner

[signature] Stephen R. Bushing   Date 9/18/2017

STEPHEN R. BUSHING - INVENTORY DISTRIBUTION CONTROL MANAGER

I certify that all information furnished on this form is true and complete. I understand that anyone who furnishes false or misleading information on this form or who omits material or information requested on the form may be subject to criminal sanctions (including fines and imprisonment) and/or civil sanctions (including civil penalties).

PS Form 3526, July 2014 [Page 1 of 4 (see instructions page 4)]   PSN: 7530-01-000-9931   PRIVACY NOTICE: See our privacy policy on www.usps.com.

PS Form 3526, July 2014 (Page 3 of 4)   PRIVACY NOTICE: See our privacy policy on www.usps.com.

Moving?

Make sure your subscription moves with you!

To notify us of your new address, find your **Clinics Account Number** (located on your mailing label above your name), and contact customer service at:

Email: journalscustomerservice-usa@elsevier.com

800-654-2452 (subscribers in the U.S. & Canada)
314-447-8871 (subscribers outside of the U.S. & Canada)

Fax number: 314-447-8029

Elsevier Health Sciences Division
Subscription Customer Service
3251 Riverport Lane
Maryland Heights, MO 63043

ELSEVIER

Printed and bound by CPI Group (UK) Ltd, Croydon, CR0 4YY

08/05/2025

01864703-0001